all night

&

*talk to him
in the morning*

Make love all night

&

talk to him in the morning

*bite-size tips
for sex and relationships*

Dr. Pam Spurr

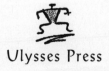

Ulysses Press

Published by Ulysses Press
            P.O. Box 3440
            Berkeley CA 94703
            www.ulyssespress.com

First published as *Sex, Guys and Chocolate* in Great Britain in 2003 by Robson Books

ISBN 1-56975-441-1
Library of Congress Control Number 2004108858

Editorial and production staff: Ashley Chase, Lee Micheaux, Pani Page
Cover photograph: arttoday.com
Cover design: Sarah Levin, Leslie Henriques
Interior design: Leslie Henriques

Printed in Canada by Transcontinental Printing

10 9 8 7 6 5 4 3 2 1

Distributed in the United States by Publishers Group West and in Canada by Raincoast Books

CONTENTS

. . . and Talk to Him in the Morning

Acknowledgements

I'd like to thank every person who has helped me with this book by sharing their life stories with me. When someone asks another person for advice this becomes a two-way process: by asking, hopefully they get something helpful from the process; but at the same time, they open the eyes of the person *giving* advice. I love talking to people about their stories because that is what life is about—each individual's story. What we forget is that we *are* the authors of our own stories. So be creative and powerful when writing yours! . . . Lastly, warm thanks to my publisher, Jeremy Robson.

Introduction

I'm continually asked for a handy little guide to relationships and sex—dating, mating and relating. We've all become so busy that creating a book you can quickly flip through for lots of answers seemed a fantastic project to get involved with. It's also a project that's close to my heart, as my work has covered so many aspects of women's sex and relationship issues. Please note I say "*lots* of the answers!" No single book can contain *all* the answers to the dilemmas we face in modern relationships, when the rules seem to change all the time. Hopefully you'll find a lot of useful advice and inspiration within the following chapters, and suggestions that may become a springboard to sorting out other issues in your life.

How did I decide what to include? Since my work as a sex advisor, life coach and psychologist has covered so many different areas, it seemed a logical step to have a good look at what most women ask about, where they get stuck, and the most common problems they face. Trawling through literally thousands of e-mails, letters and questions I've had in recent years pointed me in the right directions. The topics in *Make Love All Night... And Talk to Him in the Morning* are the sexual and romantic topics that most women have questions about, even if they just chat about them with their friends and family. Often we simply want an unbiased opinion and a constructive attitude from someone who is neutral—and that's where I've come in over the years in my various roles.

Sex has everyone confused these days. Who does what to whom? Where's my sex drive hiding? Why is my sex life so unfulfilling? How can I explain what I'd like to do in bed? Why don't I have any sexual confidence? Can I share my sexual fantasies without offending him? Many of our attitudes toward sex have changed, but too often we don't have the knowledge to keep up with our new attitudes. This leads many women to feel a lack of confidence about what they want from sexual relationships. But questions like, "How soon should I have sex?" and "How do I give good oral sex?" are not the only sorts of questions I'm asked in this area. Women want to know more about

STIs (sexually transmitted infections), new sexual techniques, Tantric and safer sex, among many other things.

When it comes to dating and relationships the boundaries are terribly blurred. We all get so many mixed messages nowadays we're left wondering—Should I ask a man out? What's the best way of flirting? How can I tell if he's attracted to me? Why hasn't he called? We may be in charge of our career and sure of our destiny, but when it comes to the age-old questions of romance we fear getting it wrong.

Even if you only want to date for fun or play the field, you want to have positive experiences that enhance your self-confidence. Later on when you want to settle down, the more positive your dating experiences have been the more positive your outlook to lasting love will be. Then you'll attract the right men!

There are so many *external* worries we have about getting into a relationship: We worry about keeping our independence and not losing our identity. Then we wonder why we can't form healthy relationships, when we've really been shying away from them! *Within* our relationships we also have considerable concerns. We wonder why we end up in an unhappy pattern of destructive relationships. We're not even sure what we want out of a relationship in the first place.

To answer all these dating and relationship questions, I've taken crucial issues and laid out straightforward advice and information supported by psychological research. Once you've met a man you want to keep, I'll help you understand how men think, feel, communicate and relate to you. I hope you can find the inspiration and information you need to improve your chances of finding and keeping love.

Two pieces of advice I received from my parents put my relationships in perspective. Shortly before my mother passed away in January 2003 she said to me, "Be as happy as you can be with your husband and family." I realized the most important thing I could do for my marriage was simply to enjoy it and put it first. My father also had advice for me before his passing in May 1999. He told me, "Grab opportunities with both hands and enjoy life!" Two very different pieces of advice, but related nonetheless. When you're at your happiest in your relationships you're most likely to grab those opportunities. And when you grab opportunities—for fun, adventure and inspiration—you'll feel happy. All of life, love and relationships are interlinked this way.

If you don't find the answer to your particular dilemma in these pages then please take a closer look at some of the organizations I've mentioned that may have further information.

Good luck with your adventures in dating, mating and relating! We only have one life—make your sexual and romantic relationships the best you can!

Make Love All Night...

Why Do You Want Sex Anyway?

Can you answer the question, "Why do you want to have sex anyway?" Right now you may be wondering why I'm asking *you* that! "Because I want to feel good Dr. Pam—Doh!" Well let me tell you that women have sex for completely different reasons. Because they want physical closeness, because they want to be loved, because they're drunk or high on drugs, because they get an emotional "high" from it, because they've been pressured into it, because they want something and they think sex may lead to it, for revenge, because they're chasing an elusive orgasm and hope to get it this time, because they simply think they should—as a young liberated woman, among many other reasons.

One of the most important rules for having good sex is knowing why you're getting into bed with someone—because this helps prevent regrets. If you've thought this far about having sex then you're more likely to go to bed with someone for the right reasons. Or at least you may know you're on a path to nowhere if your reasons are dodgy. Forewarned is forearmed. Here are some *good* reasons to have sex:

- You're in lust and confident—so you're not worried if it ends up as a one-night stand.

- You're falling for someone and now it seems right.

- You're in love and he is too.

- You've a busy life and simply need sexual gratification on your terms—and he knows what they are—no strings attached. "Fuck buddies"—as it's called!

All of these examples and other reasons are fine—*if they're fine for you* and you practice safer sex.

Play Safer!

The sexiest lovers are those who care about their sexual health—*and* that of their lover. They don't want to catch or spread sexually transmitted infections (STIs). Any potential lover you come across who will *not* use condoms is *a* simply not sexy. And *b* no one you should have sex with. In an ideal world—rather than the real world we inhabit—both of you will have condom confidence. Just in case you come across a man who doesn't feel comfortable putting on a condom—build your own condom confidence. Get a variety *free* from your primary care physician or family planning clinics. *Read the instructions first!* Open the packet carefully so that you don't damage the condom. Grip the tip of the condom to squeeze out any air. Slide it on to a vibrator, carrot, cucumber, broom handle—anything penis shaped! Voilà—it's that easy. Practice makes perfect! Male condom complaints:

- "I can't feel anything with a condom." *Solution:* Put a drop of water-based lube inside the tip of the condom to enhance his sensations, and try the "extra-sensitive" types.

- "I can't find a condom that fits." *Solution:* Try the variety available—there's one for every penis shape!

- "I want to really *feel* you!" *Solution:* Both get screened for STIs, then retested for HIV—then go for it without condoms. It'll feel *even better* once you've waited! But unless you're planning a pregnancy, use some other birth control method once you give up the condoms.

- "Condoms irritate me!" *Solution:* Use ones without Nonoxynol-9 (N-9), the spermicide that irritates some people. Many specialists in sexual health are asking for the removal of N-9 from condoms and lubricants as it's now believed it *increases* the risk of HIV infection. However, its use in spermicidal creams and gels for use with other forms of barrier contraception (sponges, suppositories, etc.) is considered safe for women at low risk of HIV infection, i.e. in relationships with men they can trust.

Safer Sex—Talking About It

You deserve sexual health so how do you start talking about it? Here are points to consider smoothing any communication along.

Where Research shows that talking about sex in the bedroom can make matters worse. The reason? If the conversation takes a negative turn, a couple may then associate the bedroom with a negative experience, clouding future sexual encounters there. Always having sex in the bedroom can get boring—but bed-sex has its place. Most people make love in their bedroom or sitting room. So choose neutral ground. Also, if you start getting hot and horny in the bedroom you may not finish the conversation!

When It is always best to talk about sex when you're not heavily under the influence of alcohol (or drugs). Alcohol loosens our inhibitions and sometimes we may say things we regret or *in a way* we regret without enough tact. Of course, a little alcohol can relax you—and that's fine.

How   Keep it simple—begin with, for example, "I want to protect myself *and you* so I want to have safer sex." If you beat about the bush your lover will think you have something to hide, or just get nervous about the whole thing if he lacks sexual confidence. You make it *easier* taking this approach. Always use a clear but relaxed tone of voice. Then simply ask, "How do you feel about this?"

Finally   If you agree, bring on the condoms! You'll already have condom confidence if you followed the previous advice above!

Preventing Sexually Transmitted Infections

So you know how to use condoms—but how do you find out more about safer sex? In addition to discussing safer sex and being screened for Sexually Transmitted Infections (STIs) by your primary care physician, the U.S. National STD Hotline (800-227-8922) provides anonymous and confidential information on STIs, how to prevent them and where to get tested. Planned Parenthood (www.planned parenthood.org) is another resource for information on STIs and provides screening services. For online information and links, visit the American Social Health Association's website at www.ashastd.org.

Within the past ten years, chlamydia rates have increased, with women having an infection rate three times higher than men (mostly because more women than men are screened for this infection). Still, incidences remain highest among women aged 19 to 24. Genital warts (HSV) continue to plague one out of five sexually-active people, while the number of new cases still climbs (remember, there is no cure for genital warts or the Herpes virus that causes them). Syphilis rates, however, are on a steady decline, while gonorrhea infections are also decreasing. Despite the drop in some infection rates, the ever-present threat of STIs remains very real.

Some STI Info to Get You Thinking

These are just a few of the nasties you might pick up.

Chlamydia A bacterium that can lay dormant for years. Symptoms include abdominal pain and vaginal discharge, among others. Scary fact—70 percent of women are symptomless.

Gonorrhea Another nasty bacterium, taking two to ten days to show symptoms, including vaginal discharge, abdominal pain, painful urination—but over 60 percent of women are symptomless.

Herpes Simplex Virus 1 and 2 HSV1 usually affects the mouth (cold sores) but sometimes the genitals, and HSV2 is the other way round. Oral sex can transmit it. You'll experience painful little clear or yellowish genital blisters. Recurrent attacks become less painful but it's a life-long problem. Treatment alleviates symptoms and you will be taught how to avoid passing the virus on.

Human Papilloma Virus (*HPV*)   This causes genital warts, which can take months to show. They may appear as "lumpiness" in the skin or as little "cauliflower" style warts. There are different treatments available.

Syphilis   Also known as the "pox," this is a spiral-shaped germ that can take from one to twelve weeks to show. There are three stages. First, a painless red spot appears, becoming ulcer like. Then you may get a skin rash and, eventually, if left untreated, leads to, for example, blindness and heart problems.

Other STIs   These include hepatitis, cystitis, bacterial vaginosis, non-specific urethritis, pelvic inflammatory disease, lice, thrush, trichomonas and others. Any symptom you experience in the genitals, abdomen and/or anal passage should be checked, as symptoms vary tremendously from person to person. Permanent damage to reproduction as well as death (syphilis) can result from leaving STIs untreated.

HIV and AIDS

The human immunodeficiency virus (HIV) multiplies within a person, living off the "host" and preventing normal function of the white blood cells that help fight infections. HIV is passed on via any exchange of body fluids, including during sex, sharing needles among drug users, and in infected breast milk. Many who worry about their sexual health probably worry about HIV infection most because of its association with its development into full-blown acquired immune deficiency syndrome (AIDS), where the body can no longer fight the variety of infections we run into in daily life. The safer sex campaigns of the eighties did lots to raise awareness but now many people seem much less concerned.

The disease is still out there and it can take three to six months for an HIV test to register an antibody reaction in your system. As there are no specific symptoms for an HIV-positive person, the disease can go undetected for as much as ten or fifteen years. And, of course, it can be passed around during this time. The first indication of infection may be when a person has difficulty fighting off minor illnesses.

If you're HIV-positive, your doctor will more than likely prescribe anti-viral drugs, along with other medicines to help you fight off minor illnesses. Overall, doctors will help plan how to keep you healthy. There are a number of sources of support for those diagnosed with HIV and/or AIDS. Call the National AIDS HotLine (800-342-2437) for further information.

Contraception

Successful contraception is only possible if used *as directed*. Contraception failures tend to occur when women don't follow instructions *to the letter*. You can get contraceptive advice at any family planning or reproductive health clinic. Planned Parenthood affiliates operate 855 health centers in 49 states, serving women and teens. To find the clinic closest to you call 800-230-7526

Contraception allows you to take control of your life and decide when (if ever) you want to have a baby. There is a wide range of contraceptive products available. When you go for a consultation you should have a full and frank discussion of your sexual health and lifestyle needs. Ask any question you wish. It's advisable to go along with a question list so you don't forget anything.

The range of contraception available includes barrier methods: the male condom, the female condom, and spermicides such as foam, cream, jelly, or suppositories deposited into the vagina; combined hormone methods: the Pill, the Ring (a small, flexible ring placed deep into the vagina for three weeks), and the Patch (placed on the skin to release hormones); and progestin-only methods: implants (placed under the skin of your upper arm to constantly release small amounts of hormone), the Shot (an injection of hormones in your arm or buttock every 12 weeks), the progestin-only birth control pill, and the IUD (intra-uterine device). Emergency contraception is now available when you're worried about contraceptive failure such as a split condom, or have had unprotected sex (the "morning after" pill may prevent pregnancy for up to 72 hours, while the IUD protects up to five days later). There's also the option of male and female sterilization.

Conception—Making Mini Yous!

Before you even start thinking about having sex *to have a baby* you should consider what creating a mini-you actually means! Many go into parenthood with rose-colored specs on thinking how wonderful it'll be to have a baby to *love them!* It's quite the reverse—babies need your love and attention a full 24/7. There's no respite unless you've got parents or friends to help.

You and your partner should think about the changes a baby will mean to your relationship. No more sleeping in or late nights, or making love when you want. Go into it having agreed what sorts of roles you two will play. But be prepared for these to be thrown to the wind once you actually become parents. Do lots of babysitting for others to give you a small taster.

Aside from these practical and emotional considerations, look at your health and lifestyle—especially the mom-to-be. If you're actually planning a pregnancy—rather than having found yourself pregnant—consult your doctor or nurse practitioner about how long you should wait after coming off birth control before trying for a baby. For example, you may be advised to wait three months to clear your system of any hormones. Start taking a folic acid supplement (400 mg daily until the twelfth week of pregnancy), stop smoking and cut down on alcohol and caffeine consumption in preparation for a healthy pregnancy. Check out the National Women's Health Information Center (www.4women.gov/pregnancy) for loads of info.

Abortion

Terminating a pregnancy is something you may or may not have to consider at some point. The most important thing, if you find yourself pregnant and it's unplanned, is to seek help so you can talk through your options. The longer you wait to seek help, the more difficult your choice may be. If you leave your pregnancy longer than 20 weeks, you will most likely not qualify for an abortion unless there is a serious risk to your health.

The Supreme Court has held that women have the constitutional right to choose an abortion before the time when a fetus is viable, or could survive outside the womb (about 20-22 weeks). However, abortion rights are under constant challenge, and medical advances continue to push the time of viability earlier and earlier. Access to abortion in the second and third trimesters is more limited and tightly regulated by certain states. Almost 90 percent of abortions in the U.S. occur in the first trimester, with only 5 percent being performed after 16 weeks.

Abortions within the first trimester are either medical or surgical. A medical abortion can be performed within the first 63 days of pregnancy and is non-invasive, meaning the pregnancy is ended with pills or a shot with a follow-up pill. A surgical abortion, however, is an invasive procedure and can be done anytime during the first trimester. Planned Parenthood (www.plannedparenthood.org) can help you decide which one is best. Remember, abortion laws frequently change and vary by state, while the procedure faces routine legal objection.

Whether or not your health insurance covers an abortion depends upon the plan and provider. Your best bet is to contact your health care provider.

The Look of Lust—How to Tell
If He Likes You

Male body language is fairly obvious, hence the infamous Mae West quote, "Is that a pistol in your pocket or are you just pleased to see me?" Well, you may not see an erection but look out for the following when you lock eyes on him:

The double take   He spots you, looks away but can't resist going back for a second look rather quickly. This is a dead give away—unless you've got a massive spot on your nose that he can't take his eyes off!

He only has eyes for you   Even if a gorgeous girl walks past he barely notices. His glances keep going in your direction.

His posture   He pulls himself up so he's standing straight and he may link his fingers into his belt loop in a subconscious gesture to draw your eyes to his manhood.

He smiles!   A simple smile speaks volumes—he wants a smile back!

His walk   He begins to saunter that masculine walk.

The small talk   He gets talking to you—it may even be about something inane—so talk back. Ask him a question to keep the conversation flowing.

The bridge   He touches your forearm as he speaks to you, bringing your personal spaces together.

The block   He moves so that his upper body is blocking you from the rest of the bar/nightclub/whatever—literally blocking off any competition from locking eyes on you.

"Check me out"   He keeps looking over at the guys for approval to say "check out my success." He really likes you—or his chances!

Sexual Confidence—Know Thyself

The first step to sexual confidence is finding out how your body works. This is crucial. There should be no shame in exploring your own sexual responses through masturbation. One research survey found 98 percent of men said they had masturbated, while only 75 percent of women said they had. Some weren't telling the truth, of course, but sadly too many women I come across have a fear of touching or looking at their own body—even in our modern times.

"Mirror, mirror" Get a mirror, lie back and simply look at your genitals. Examine every little inch of your vagina, labia, clitoris, anus and perineum (the area between the vulva and the anus). The more you look the more comfortable you'll feel.

Tender touch Ensure you're comfortable. If you haven't masturbated before, start by caressing your breasts, arms, abdomen and thighs—anywhere you can reach that feels good! You can do this sitting or lying comfortably, or in the bath or shower. Use some massage oil or lubricant to heighten sensations. If you really have a problem about touching your genitals, you may first want to touch yourself through your panties to build confidence. Caress yourself slowly. Enjoy the sensations. Build to fully touching yourself as your excitement increases. This is a good, healthy thing to do. It's not "dirty" or "sordid"—so don't let anyone tell you that!

Keep this in mind. Women are NOT mind readers, and men are even worse! How can your lover guess how to give you pleasure if you won't even learn about your own responses?

Sexual Confidence II—
Building to Orgasm

The female orgasm—or climax—is complicated. Only about 20 percent of women regularly climax through penetrative sex with their partners. Most need to use a combination of stimulation—hands, oral sex, sex toys and so on, to help them on their way during sex. Depending on the study, some 15 percent or so of women never climax during penetrative sex.

So, by learning how to bring yourself to orgasm through masturbation, you can then put this knowledge to good use with a lover—and recreate the sensations you know work for you. This means lots of experimenting when you're not in a rush. Now that you've experienced pleasurable sensations during masturbation it may still take you some exploring to find out how to get all the way to orgasm.

Feel free to try different things. For example, some women find they can only climax by using the palm of their hand, or by rubbing against a pillow or cushion. Others like to introduce a vibrator or dildo (a penis-shaped sex toy that doesn't vibrate) to help them on their way. This is where Frank Sinatra comes in handy—live by his saying, "I did it my way" and you can't go wrong!

Some women experience orgasm as a slow build-up of sexual tension with a powerful release that may come in waves. Others experience a quick build-up with a short release. Still others feel a much more gentle form of sensual experience. On average, an orgasm lasts about 6–8 seconds. Keep in mind what works for you—for example, vigorous finger stimulation or a gentle rubbing—to teach your lover.

Sexual Confidence III—
You're a Love and Sex Goddess

Visualizations work! Cancer patients who visualize strong white blood cells cleaning up their systems have been found to have an increased production of these important cells. Those who visualize for academic work can achieve scores 10 percent higher. And athletes who visualize their last great goal are more likely to score another. It's all about gaining a positive mindset. So *you* can visualize being a love goddess!

Get comfortable *in* something really sexy—feeling that you *look* sexy will help you visualize yourself as a sex goddess. Recline in a big armchair or easy chair where you're warm enough in your slinky little negligée. Close your eyes and take a few relaxing breaths. Feel your breasts move up and down gently with your breathing. Allow your legs to relax and your hands to flop by your sides, unless you wish to touch yourself.

Now visualize someone you think of as being really sexy—maybe an icon like Marilyn Monroe, or someone in the news right now. Run your eyes over her image. What makes her sexy and sensuous? What are her qualities? Maybe she's just gorgeous and voluptuous. Maybe she's got real character. What you think counts.

Now imagine yourself having those qualities—you lolling about loving every inch of your sensual self. Place this image on a pedestal surrounded by sex slaves pandering to your every whim. You are this gorgeous amazing sex goddess. Affirm to yourself that you are *worthy* of great sex. Hold this image each day for a few moments.

A Big Secret
To Boost Your Confidence Further

He's as worried as you are! He's cute, he's in between your
sheets and you're having a panic attack in the bathroom
thinking you're going to let him down in bed—your sexual confidence has plummeted to a big fat zero! Well guess
what—that hunk warming your sheets is just as worried
about having sex with you! Having spoken to thousands
of men in my role as agony aunt and life coach, 99.9 percent worry about the first time they sleep with you. They
are saying to themselves "Will I be too fast?" "Will I lose
my erection?" (two of the most common male sexual fears)
and "Will her ex-lovers be better then me?" So relax—you
both may be a bundle of nerves—this is human. Taking it
slowly will help you feel (literally!) your way through your
first lovemaking session. It's not a competition to see who's
more experienced. It's about getting to know each other.

So how do you do this? You undress each other
slowly—unless it's one of those hot *just-in-the-door-rip-*

each-other's-clothes-off-and-do-it-standing-up jobs! And that means you're both sexually confident. Take time lingering over his buttons or zips. Build this into foreplay. Make his heart skip a few beats by allowing this time to build up.

Give him the confidence to take his time with you, too. Whisper that you're not in a rush and you want to take it slowly. Sometimes women have to take charge of building this sort of confidence. Go for it—you'll both have a better time leading to increased sexual confidence!

Developing Your Sex Muscles

You can greatly enhance your sex life and genital health by exercising your sex muscles—the pubococcygeal (PC, or "pelvic floor") muscles. Research has found that the strength and tone of these muscles contribute to sexual pleasure and orgasmic capability in women. And in men, exercising PC muscles can contribute greatly to learning how to control their ejaculatory response—that is, they can last longer. How do you identify your PC muscles? Think about when you're peeing and you want to stop the flow of urination. These are the muscles that allow you to do that. The best way to exercise them is to start at a low level and build slowly.

Begin with ten repetitions, twice a day. To begin with, you may wish to get comfortable sitting, lying or standing. But once you've mastered this you'll find you can do your exercises at your desk, on the bus, anywhere. Even during sex—your lover will love the pulsing sensation as you clamp and unclamp your PC muscles. A repetition consists of tightening and holding for a count of two or three. As you gain control of your PC muscles you can build to twenty repetitions three times a day. After doing your repetitions, stroke your PC muscles and the surrounding area to relax them, running your strokes from either side of your clitoris, down the sides of your labia, to your perineum.

The benefits of a strong pelvic floor include better orgasms as well as prevention of bladder weakness (or improvement if you already have the problem). This is particularly important after pregnancy.

Developing Your Sex Muscles—Level II

Build your vaginal muscle strength by other inventive means. Ever thought of weight training with your vagina? You can—by using weights attached to a love "egg" or ball. These weights can be put in a cloth bag and strung on to the little safety "pull string" that love "eggs" have. Or purchase solid "eggs" on the Internet with an "eye" to string the weights through.

     Stage one simply involves working the inner vaginal muscles to hold the "egg" in place. Start with a larger "egg" and work down to smaller ones—this is even harder as you have to "hang on" to them! Remember to clean any "eggs" purchased thoroughly by disinfecting and then boiling. Next, use small weights (beware of any hooks!) bagged and attached to the "egg." Start with 6–9 oz (175–250 g) and ensure you don't overuse your inner muscles. Slowly build up the weight you use.

Instead of "eggs," try *standing* and gripping a vibrator (when it's turned off, obviously!), if you have one, as it's a harder shape to hold on to than an "egg." Next, begin to crouch slowly and see how far you can crouch before your muscles let the vibrator slip.

Finally, why not go for a bit of a flutter. Once your pelvic floor muscles are stronger you'll find that not only can you contract and release them anywhere, any time, but you can flutter them. Imagine the way a belly dancer rolls her stomach—try this with your pelvic floor.

The Best Sex

You can settle for OK sex but I hope you want more. I'm not talking now about technique and choosing crazy sexual positions or the weirdest stuff you can do without being classified as a raving pervert. I'm talking about simply enjoying sex on *your* terms. Having spoken to thousands of women, there seem to be two criteria for deciding how much good or bad sex they're getting. These are: when they wait long enough (*see* "One-Night Stands" on page 136) to feel they can *communicate* with their lover, and when they feel in *control*.

Communication first   Think about this—if you're only just getting to know a man and wouldn't feel comfortable discussing your mother's alcoholism, your uncle's depression or a recent humiliation at work—how on earth can you discuss sex and likes/dislikes/fantasies/and so on? If you can't discuss it, how will it be safer and enjoyable?

Too many women close their eyes (not literally but metaphorically!) hoping for the best—not daring to say anything to a new lover about sex. Not good! If you wait until you can talk about it before having sex it'll be better sex—I guarantee it.

Next there's *control* You'll have far better sex if you're in control. By control I mean—when you want it, in a place you want it and how you want it. The simple rule? Don't have it *until you want it*. You know you're going to enjoy it as you're not sneaking behind parents' or roommates' backs, and you feel absolutely ready.

Before-play

Before-play is a concept I first introduced into sex advice about five years ago. After speaking to vast numbers of women—especially those who'd lost desire—I realized that there wasn't enough good stuff going on *before* sex to put them in the mood to even start. So I coined the term "before-play" to remind people of the importance of how you feel *generally* in your life and about the man in your life, and the effect this has on how sexy you feel. This is just as important with a new lover as one you've been with for a long time.

If you both have loads of stress in your life, are edgy being in a new relationship with each other (maybe due to past "baggage') or have just argued—you won't be in the mood for sex (although some couples adore make-up sex!). So never forget the principles of romance, respect and generally having lots of goodwill for each other and the role it plays in making you feel sexy.

If, for example, your long-term lover has just forgotten your birthday, or your new man is more interested in himself than you, then you will not feel very sexy. He'll feel the same way if you neglect him. Before the first hint of foreplay begins, make romantic gestures, be affectionate, see the good in each other and generally care for each other—and sex will stay alive for you!

Getting What You Want

The women who get what they want in bed have the sexual confidence to communicate and take control, and are also good at the *give and take* of great sex. Let's begin with "*taking*" first—more fun! There are many ways of getting a man to pleasure you. These are the most effective:

- Men love to be asked! Use a sexy and seductive voice and *ask* him for what you want. If you preface this by saying, "*I know you'll be so good at it* so will you please dribble this massage oil over my buttocks and swirl it around" you'll have him on his knees dying to do it for you!

- Show him how to do it! For example, if you love your nipples being sucked in a particular way, then suck his in that way, look up at him with a naughty smile and say, "Will you suck my nipples like that, too?" Or, take his finger (or even his penis!) and suck it with the pressure and style you love and say, "It'd feel fantastic if you sucked my nipples like this!"

• Use pictures! Take his favorite men's mag—or your girl's mag—or a sex guide like my book *Naughty Tricks and Sexy Tips*, and show him a photo, article or passage that describes what you'd like to do.

• Move him into position! You can always take his hand, his head (!), his penis and so on, and move it to where you want it, creating the action that turns you on.

Giving Him What He Wants

Just as it's rewarding for you to get good "technique" given to you—so it's rewarding to give him what he wants. Many women think it's "slutty" to be too good in bed—not true! You'll both be happier if you know that your lover's satisfied. Try these most effective methods:

- Ask him what he wants! You'll not be seen as a scarlet woman if you whisper, "What would you like me to do" as you run your fingers down his chest. No, he'll see you as a Sex Goddess straight from heaven and will eagerly tell you his likes.

- Experiment and listen to his sex noises! Try different techniques and simply listen to his responses. Unless he's "Mr. Silent-type," men let slip little noises that tell you whether or not you're hitting the spot. So stay tuned to his sex sounds.

- Describe a sex scene to him! Telling him about something you think he'll like can have two effects: *1* you'll hit it on the button and it's something he likes too, or *2* you'll introduce him to something new. So if you love the "feeding frenzy" between Mickey Rourke and Kim Bassinger in *9½ Weeks* say, "It'd be fantastic to drip cream down your chest and between your thighs to lick off gently!"

- Map out his erogenous zones! Tell him you're on a mission of discovery. With a feather, basting brush, end of a whip—trace all around his body, asking what feels best—and remember his answers!

Feeling Sexy—Your Timing and His

Depending on your own sexual "clock" you may feel horniest during ovulation (when your body says it's time to make babies), or just before your period, owing to hormonal changes, or, for some women, after their period, when they feel calm and in control. Men also peak at different times as their testosterone levels change—often over a 24-hour period. Some are morning-men—others are naughty at night.

When sleeping with each other for the first time, you may both feel like having sex all the time. But it's quite natural for things to settle down after three to six months. At this point, your essential levels of sex drive may determine whether or not you experience problems in this department. Many couples find that one or the other "*feels like it*" more frequently than the other. You *can* sort this out.

First, when the first flush of lust starts to dwindle, neither of you should take it personally—talk about it. Second, it's critical to keep the romance going (so neither of you feels neglected) as well as building in a few new sex tricks to keep things lively *when you do have sex*. Next, take turns initiating sex so you both feel you're keeping things alive. It's easy for the one with a higher sex drive to do all the initiating—this can get annoying. Finally, if there are big differences in your sex drives, ask: is sex being used to play out other difficulties? Is one of you overworked, stressed or ill?

Blissful Kissing

Your lips are so packed with nerve endings, research shows that even a gentle brush across them can stimulate an area in the brain larger than the one stimulated by a touch to your genitals! Your lips also swell slightly and deepen in colour when you're attracted to someone or sexually aroused. Kissing is incredibly intimate, which is why many prostitutes will do everything *but!*

The first kiss: if you'd like to kiss him but aren't sure if he wants to, simply move in closer, ensure your head is tilted up to his and speak in soft tones. This'll increase his kissing confidence. Many women (and men!) worry about how to kiss a man. Here are some tips for a sensational smooch:

1. practice on the *inside* of your wrist to gauge what your lips feel like when in kissing mode.

2. Check out your oral hygiene—is your breath fresh?

3. Loosen your lips as you go in for the kill. Tight lips are a turn-off!

4. Allow your tongue to relax too—only use it in a stiff poking kiss with the suggestions below. Let it swirl around the inside of his lips and the roof of his mouth (both neglected places that feel great when gently stimulated) as well as circling his tongue with yours.

5. Just go with the moment—it may be a gentle or passionate kiss but people who really like each other have a subconscious way of getting there in the end—even if their noses bump at first!

Advanced Kissing

A few advanced kissing techniques can turn you into a great lover. Here are some favorites to try.

The Medieval Necklet   Encircle the delicate skin on your lover's neck with little kisses. Start behind his ear and plant wet little kisses, making a circle that goes down his collar bone, ending up behind his other ear.

The Vacuum   Allow your lips to relax then encircle your lover's closed lips. Gently apply a little sucking—or vacuum—to his outer lips and pulsate slowly. You are in control. The delicate skin around his lips will be stimulated and feel fantastic.

The Snake   As the name suggests, you ease your tongue across your lover's lips, into his mouth and *anywhere* on his body in little flicking motions. Great for flicking little crumbs of food off his body after food-play.

These are techniques to ask your lover to try on you:

The Naughty Dog This passionate, earthy kiss is great for larger erogenous zones like the whole breast, abdomen and inner thigh. Ask your lover to start at the base of your breast and lap upward, flicking your nipple as he finishes the lap. He can use it on the inner thigh, finishing the lap with a gentle flick, going down your inner thigh toward the knee or up toward the genitals.

The Eastern Swirl and Poke Originating in the Far East, this feels heavenly. Ask your lover to use it with a French kiss or on your body. He first swirls around with his tongue encircling yours, then pokes gently with the tip of his tongue. This feels great on the nipples, around the belly button and genitals.

Oral Sex—Getting Started

Oral sex is a deeply intimate act that can give enormous pleasure, but it can also create great anxiety. Men and women worry about giving *and receiving* oral sex. Their concerns usually involve fear about how to do it and personal hygiene—will *they* like the taste of their lover—or will their lover like the way *they* taste?

Hygiene   Good hygiene's essential for you both. A bit of water play (*see page 84*) can get you both *fresh* in a sensual way. But if it's not convenient to have a bath/shower together, wash on your own before lovemaking, or introduce a warm, wet face cloth to carefully wash each other as part of foreplay. Don't forget that many women are sensitive to commercial douches/soaps/shower gels, which, ironically, can lead to irritation and a smell.

Safer oral   You can transfer nasty bugs between the mouth and the genitals. Herpes Simplex I of the mouth can be passed to the genitals and Herpes Simplex II can be carried from the genitals to the mouth. If you don't know his sexual history, use flavored condoms and give him a blow job through them. He should cover you with a dental dam/cling wrap and give you "head" through that.

Get your tongue ready   Your tongue/lips should be in shape to give all sorts of sensations. Each day, flick your tongue up and down to build its strength. Then circle it round and round. Practice swirling your lips around one of your fingers so you know what it'll feel like on the tip of his glans.

Oral Sex II—Getting It from Him

Tongue techniques

There are all sorts of tongue techniques he can use on
you. Ask him to kiss, flick and lick down your abdomen,
across your mons pubis, down either side of your labia
and your inner thighs. Not coming into contact with your
clitoris will leave you panting for more.

Nose and lips   If you have a sensitive clitoris, ask
him to use his lips and nose (yes!) to gently stimulate you.
Ask him *not* to draw back your clitoral hood, too. By
placing your hands behind his ears you can control the pressure he uses.

Loving the pearl   When you're aroused, guide him
to put his thumb and forefinger on either side of your clitoris and *gently* rub it—lots of lubricant will make this
heavenly!

V for victory   If you don't like clitoral stimulation, this is an alternative way to make you climax. He makes a "V" sign and slips his two fingers, palm down, on either side of your clit, pointing down your labia. He can then gently circle his "V" sign, arousing all the nerve endings around your mons pubis, clitoris and labia.

Finger work   Take his fingers and place them where you want, to show him the pressure you like near your clitoris. He can "drum" lightly, rub in circular motions, twirl your labia or around the clitoral region to give you wonderful sensations.

Come on over   Perfect for him to stimulate your G-spot while sucking your labia or clitoris. With palm upward, ask him to insert his index and middle fingers inside your vagina. Then he does a gentle "come here" gesture—repeatedly.

Oral Sex III—Giving It to Him

Mouth Magic

You can lap, suck, flick and tease with your tongue and lips. Ask how the different sensations feel! Practice on a penis-shaped vibrator (switched off!) to build your confidence. Get him to "direct" you.

Swirling Perfect for around the penile glans, swirling is sensual and loving. Ensure your tongue stays loose as, with a leisurely pace, you swirl lightly. You may wish to increase the pressure of your tongue as his arousal increases.

Snaking Hold your tongue loosely and allow it to slip sideways back and forth quite quickly. This feels amazing early in oral play with its gentle sweeping sensation. Start at the lower abdomen, then move down to his genitals.

Funneling   Imagine you're savoring a LifeSavers candy. Holding the imaginary LifeSavers in front of your mouth, you curl your tongue like a funnel, slipping it in and out of the hole in the center. Funneling can be used on men who like the opening of their urethra stimulated.

Humming   While holding either his glans or a testicle in your mouth hum gently—he'll love the vibes!

Hand and mouth   Use your hands, too. If your mouth tires, switch to using both hands—one at the base of his penis, one at the tip. Move them in and out first toward, and then away from each other.

Deep throat   Many women never get past the gag reflex. Your throat should be lined up straight with your jaw (head back) propped by pillows.

And finally   If you hate giving "head" kiss *around* his genitals. Or spread your favorite topping (jam, chocolate) over him and eat it off. Don't be pressured into any sex act you dislike!

Touch

Most people don't realize how many different sensations they can give and receive by simply changing the way they touch. Even changing from touching your lover with your right hand, to using your left hand will vary the sensations.

Try bringing the scalp alive with a few gentle touches to the earlobe, then circling behind the neck as you two kiss. As you touch your lover, listen to his love sounds—be guided. If he enjoys something, don't feel you have to move on. We're all in such a rush for the genitals! Don't be! Linger over what feels good to him. A big rule to remember—at different times you'll both want different areas touched. Spoil each other by taking turns touching different parts. One of you lies back while the other tickles, teases, scratches and swirls their fingers over the other's body.

Other things to try Trickle some lubricant down his stomach and swirl a feather through it. For a firmer touch, drag a clean kitchen basting brush through the lube. Why not wear some soft gloves or latex ones with lots of lube to stimulate each other? Run a vibrator over his well-lubricated skin. Keep your nails clean and short, unless he loves a scratching sensation. Check this out—some men hate being scratched!

Don't forget Inside the wrists, behind the knees, across the ankles, stroking individual toes, massaging the hands, caressing around and down the ribs. Swish your fingers back and forth, up and down the inner thighs and buttocks.

New Sexual Thrills—
Developing Your Sexth Sense!

Listen to your lover. He may drop hints. Sometimes one of you might suggest something the other's turned off by—like anal sex. This doesn't mean one of you is a "perve" and the other a prude—no judgments please, or you'll both be wary of suggesting new things.

Balloons The challenge here is for him to thrust while keeping the balloons between you—without popping them.

Jet stream Using a balloon, control a thin stream of air across your lover's lubed-up body—this feels fantastic on the genitals.

Ice and wax play Alternate sensations—first trail ice over his skin with your fingers or between your lips. Then drop a little melted wax from *one yard*—testing first on the inside of your wrist. WARNING—You or your lover can get burnt if you're not careful! You're responsible for testing the wax! Or dribble warm water over the spot you've just iced. Ensure the water is a comfortable temperature.

Stripping   Take turns stripping for each other. Practice on your own, then turn down the lights, put on some mood music and bump and grind slowly. You'll either get very turned on or laugh—both are good!

Al fresco *and other places*   Be careful of outdoor sex in your backyard if it is overlooked. Make *al fresco* sex as risky and fun as you want. Find a truly deserted beauty spot, or slip out of a party into the toilet to have a quickie!

Spanking and whipping   Start gently and move across his flesh—you don't want bruising—or do you!? Try a satin sash or cloth belt before moving up to leather.

Sex Positions

Guess what? Research shows couples stick to two or three favorites—because it's easy. But down the line it gets boring, such as sticking to "spoons" on Friday night. A few worth trying:

Spoons   Lying side by side, he penetrates from behind.

Doggy   He is behind while she is on all fours, facing down.

The spinner   He's on his back, she sits astride him and eases around first 90 degrees, so that she's sides on, then 180 degrees so that her back's to him. She controls thrusting. If he's an "ass man" he'll love the view.

The double header   He can push himself up from *the spinner* and they continue with her back pressed into his chest. Or he sits back against the sofa or headboard and she slips on to his lap with her back to his chest. A gentle "ride."

The sling   Standing with him supported by a wall, facing each other, she moves a leg up over his arm, so that it forms a "sling," and gives better access for penetrating her.

The ploughman   She's on her back, legs up, knees bent into his chest. He balances on his feet while crouching and holds her buttocks, bringing them to meet his thrusts. He can lean his hands into the bed or floor (or wherever they are!).

The puppet   He stands behind her. She bends forward like a limp puppet and either rests her hands on a bed or sofa, or, if flexible, on the floor. This gives him great G-spot access. Don't forget the "U" and "A" spots. The "U" is located just below the clitoris and above the urethral opening. The "A" (*anterior fornix*) is deeper in the vagina, past the "G."

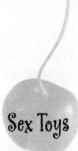

Sex Toys

Lovers should use sex toys together more often. They're fun, feel good and add to your lovemaking in many ways. And even though many women use vibrators they often hide this fact from the men in their lives. For hygiene, keep separate "his" and "her" bags of sex toys and clean them as instructed.

Men love the idea of playing with toys—but they're also a bit shy about admitting this. So start with something non-threatening, such as a small vibrator. If you thrust one of those huge vibrators in his face he'll *a* be very ashamed of his penis size and *b* find the device hard to handle! Some great toys on the market include:

Penis-shaped vibrator Have fun vibrating up and down your nipples, abdomen, perineum—and his!

Jessica Rabbit or *Pearl Rabbit vibrator*　These have "ears" to stimulate the clitoris during penetration with the vibrator.

G-spot, clit-tickler, fingertip and *bullet-style vibrators*　These are usually designed as flexible wands with vibrating ends to hit the spot.

Anal vibrators/butt plugs　For those of you willing to try something new.

Tongue Joy　A mini-vibrator that slips on your lover's tongue to give you joy everywhere he kisses you!

Vibrating cushion　He sits on it—she sits astride him and during penetration the vibrations come up between them.

Penile shaft sleeves　A huge variety of soft and flexible sleeves can be worn on finger or penis. They have bumps for extra stimulation.

Check out www.goodvibes.com

Sexy Feasts and Aphrodisiacs

Sliding between the sheets with a few pieces of chocolate, to warm up and smooth over erogenous zones, or enjoying a whole sexy feast in bed, is incredibly sensual. We forget that our mouths are centers of eroticism—be creative! Slip morsels of food into your lover's mouth. Hold a ripe strawberry dipped in cream between your lips and share. Here are some fabulous foods/additives that seem sexy and may have aphrodisiac properties:

Almonds   These contain properties said to revive flagging desire. Mediterranean cultures bake them into savories and desserts as love-symbols.

Asparagus   Hand-feed your lover warm spears dripping with melted butter.

Bananas   These give energy and contain alkaloids with aphrodisiac effects. Bake with sugar and spices, and spoon-feed your lover.

Chocolate   This contains phenylethylamine and caffeine, which stimulate the brain, and sugar, which boosts energy.

Ginger, cinnamon and ginseng powders   The Chinese have used ginger as a stimulant for 3,000 years. Eastern cultures use cinnamon and ginseng for the same purpose—bake or sprinkle on to food.

Oysters and other seafood   These contain zinc, which is beneficial for energy levels—and they look so sexy!

Avena sativa   Buy in extract form and add to food and drinks. This seems to help those with low testosterone.

Damania   A popular aphrodisiac grown in hot climates and purchased in capsule or tincture forms, it contains alkaloids that boost circulation.

Gingko biloba   Known to increase blood and oxygen flow.

Muira puama   Popular in Germany—this can be brewed or taken as a capsule.

Yohimbine   This may increase male libido, possibly by boosting neurotransmitters.

WARNING: Don't take any supplements without consulting your doctor first.

Sexual Fantasies

About 95 percent of men and 75 percent of women own up to having some sort of sexual fantasy life. I actually think it's about 98 percent ACROSS THE BOARD! Only a few people are so sexually inhibited or uninterested that their minds don't wander into sexual territory from time to time. Many women are simply embarrassed to admit to having them. Why? Because women still worry it makes them seem "slutty." This is ridiculous. Having sexual fantasies is great!

Relish these quiet moments as they may prove to be a fertile ground for spicing up your sex life. The human mind is constantly asking, "What if?" We wouldn't have evolved to the supposedly "civilized" people we are if our minds weren't always dreaming up new things to try. So, when it comes to sexual *"What ifs?"*—such as, "What if my boss threw me across the photocopier and ravished me?," "What if my neighbor caught me in the nude?" or

"What if that sexy doctor gave me an intimate examination?"—they can generate all sorts of shared fantasies and role plays. Top female fantasizes include power themes—dominating a man, being powerless, sex with strangers and lesbian sex.

Believe it or not, men find it terribly exciting to fantasize about what *you might be fantasizing* about! Men seem to think we're so complicated when many of our fantasizes are as earthy and basic as theirs. The important thing to remember is how to let them in on your naughty little fantasy life . . . coming next!

Etiquette for Sharing Your Fantasies and Other Desires

Here are half a dozen rules for sharing your fantasies:

1. Always introduce your fantasy life gently—don't storm in with, "I only get turned on thinking about having a threesome!" So, for example, if "three-way" is your fantasy, start with, "Have you ever wondered what it'd be like to have a threesome?"

2. Always clarify that this is fantasy time—not something you want to make into a reality! Do not be pressured by a partner into turning fantasy chat into a reality.

3. Always praise your partner first—this is something that'll come up repeatedly in smoothing the path of your relationships. Think of something your lover does that genuinely turns you on. For example, say, "I love it when you stroke the

backs of my thighs and buttocks, it makes me imagine that I'm lying down, sunbathing on a beach and you don't know me and you walk up and start rubbing suntan lotion into my back, buttocks and legs . . .." Then you've built a compliment straight into a fantasy.

4. If it turns out that your particular fantasy kink is a real turn-off for your lover, find another one that won't make him feel uneasy. Feeling pressured to share a fantasy can actually end up ruining your sex life.

5. Once you are both confident enough to chat about your fantasy lives, build in some role play. For example, if you're both turned on by a "stranger sex" fantasy, then meet up in a bar as "strangers in the night" and get carried away.

6. The power of fantasy can't be underestimated. When you are comfortable sharing these desires it'll liven things up—and that's what we want!

Water Play

Water is sexy—gushing, surging, splashing—it frees you up! But many women feel a little uncomfortable about what could happen during water play—how will we actually *do it*? You don't have to go "all the way" if your bath or shower is small. But you can still have fun.

Start by using candles to light your bathroom so that it looks really seductive. Turn on some mood music. You could start water play by leading your partner into the bath and simply offer to wash him or give him a back massage. This way you can slowly get into the mood to try other things. If you have a removable showerhead use it to spray him (and he you) gently from neck to toes. But don't let him spray the shower directly up into your vagina as, in *rare* circumstances, you may blast an air bubble into the bloodstream.

Lather each other up with a bath or shower gel that neither of you is allergic to (don't forget your genitals may

84

get irritated when using some products). Take turns simply washing each other's shoulders and breasts with loads of lather. Introduce one of the new waterproof sex toys to your water play—water plus vibrations feels fab! The "water duck" is definitely good fun. Beware—you can't use condoms in the bath or shower. So, if you want to use a condom, gently towel each other down—this can be incredibly sensual with big warm, fluffy towels—and then head for the bedroom.

Finally, rub lots of moisturizer or lube slowly into each other's skin. A sensual massage finishes off water play perfectly.

All Tied Up

Many people find the idea of some "vanilla" bondage a real turn on. "Vanilla" means a gentle, fairly straight, non-threatening sort of sexual activity. There are seven points to consider when thinking about introducing a little bondage play into your sex life:

1. Talk about it first. Maybe while changing your clothes, you can ask your lover to let you tie his tie. Use this opportunity to say, "Wow, it'd be cool if we put this tie to another use—like on your wrists or mine!"

2. If he seems agreeable and not shocked, next time you make love have a tie handy by the bedside, or wherever you are. Or, if your lover doesn't wear ties, then use a bathrobe belt.

3. Always tie with "bows" not knots—I can't tell you how many novices have got themselves all

tied up in knots and it's taken the pleasure out of the "event."

4. Tie loosely enough to ensure that your lover doesn't feel threatened.

5. Agree on a word that actually means you want to "stop." In the heat of the moment you may say something like, "Stop! Stop!" as part of the fantasy play, so choose a neutral word, then your lover knows you're serious.

6. Never leave anyone tied up. Don't tie each other up if you've been drinking excessively or taking drugs.

7. Build up a bedside bondage bag of goodies. Things like handcuffs, different restraints or blindfolds. Get some bondage sheets with Velcro wrist/ankle straps!

Check out www.theerogenouszone.com

Your Sex Treasure Chest

A big complaint I hear from women is that there's never anything new in their lovemaking. It's—get into position, do it and roll over. If you want to make your sex life more spontaneous you have to do some planning. That way, when you two are feeling horny, you've got a selection of playthings to suit your mood. Stock up a lockable (if you have children) chest by the bed for all your goodies. This should include:

- Lubricants and massage oils. If using condoms, only use water-based lubricants or those specifically safe for condoms. Also, don't allow oils to get inside the vagina—they can irritate your delicate pH balance.

- Your favorite sex toys, such as handcuffs, vibrators and "clit" ticklers. Store them in "his" and "hers" bags to keep them extra hygienic.

- A soft, satiny blindfold and sexy dice for sex games.

- Your favorite erotica to read to each other, or erotic films to watch together.

- Soft ties or stockings for bondage play and dressing up.

- A feather or basting brush for touching techniques.

- Condoms, dental dams, cling wrap and latex gloves for safer sex play—if you don't know your partner's sexual history.

- Erotic edibles—chocolates and honey don't need refrigeration and are perfect for sex play.

- Your favorite mood music CD so it's not lost among the rest of your music colle time is right.

- A box of luxury tissues—need I say

Check out www.mypleasure.com

Forbidden Practices—
Anal Sex for Him and Her

Anal sex has been practiced by various cultures throughout history. The enlightened Sumerians practiced hetero- and homosexual anal sex. Often anal sex was used to give pleasure without fear of pregnancy. That said, many still have a taboo about such "forbidden" practices. Explore this tactfully with your lover. No one should feel pressured into anal sex if they're put off by it. However, anal sex is not advisable unless you know your partner's sexual history as there is an increased risk of HIV transmission. Always use a condom, avoiding those that contain the spermicide N-9.

- The rectum needs to be emptied, naturally or with a suppository.

- Expel any wind first—going to the bathroom, getting on all fours and tilting your bottom upward helps! This'll prevent some embarrassing noises.

- Ensure your anal area and hands are clean.

- Relaxation is incredibly important. Tension means the outer sphincter won't relax, causing pain. Foreplay should help with arousal and relaxation of the anal area.

- Use lots of water-based lubricant. Unlike the vagina, the anal passage is not naturally lubricated. Re-apply generously!

- Try simple touching and then gentle partial finger penetration (wearing latex gloves) to stimulate this delicate area. Trim your nails for finger play!

- To get started, try inserting one latex-gloved finger into the anus. Keep it still, allowing the sphincter to relax.

- Build to penetration with the penis, anal vibrator, or strap-on—for the man who wants to be penetrated! The person being penetrated should control the depth and speed of thrusting.

- Individuals have different tastes in terms of positions. Some prefer "spoons," others "doggy" and others the "double header" (*see page 74*).

When He's Too Quick

Men have complicated feelings about sex. Yes, when it suits them (one-night stands!) they can switch off emotionally and totally enjoy a physical moment. But their sense of worth is bound up in their performance. Many dread one of two problems: coming too quickly—premature ejaculation (PE)—and losing their erection (*see page 94*). Men frequently experience PE out of sheer excitement, especially when having "first-time" sex with someone new (90 percent of men have reported this happening with at least one partner). Other men get into a habit of PE (often learned as a teen when they rushed for fear of discovery) that they find hard to break. These six steps will help a man who is experiencing PE:

1. Encourage him to build his PC muscle (*see page 46*) then . . .

2. Through masturbation, he identifies his "point of no return"—where he *has* to ejaculate. Before

this point is the plateau stage. This is where developing stronger PC muscles helps. As he reaches his "point," some simple squeezes of the PC muscles will help him to stop ejaculating.

3. He should introduce this new control gradually into lovemaking.

4. During lovemaking, he can concentrate on your sensations first—building his confidence.

5. Use positions that give less friction during penetration. This'll also help him control his PE. In these positions he can stimulate you with his hand or a sex toy.

6. For some men, "second time around" is much slower and, as well as practicing the above, he may be happy to have a second, slower go!

When His Erection Fails

One in ten men experience erectile dysfunction (ED) at some point in their life. According to the National Institutes of Health, 15 to 30 million men in the United States experience chronic ED. Usually it is transitory but it rocks a man's confidence to the core if it happens. It may occur in response to a heavy drinking session or drug taking or as a side-effect of medicine or a physical disorder, such as diabetes. It can also be emotional.

If he can get and maintain an erection during masturbation, or if he wakes with a morning erection, then the problem is likely to be emotional. For example, he feels threatened in the relationship, or it is in response to a lifestyle choice—perhaps he drinks heavily at night and then can't "get it up."

Encourage your partner to masturbate and experiment privately with his erection. This can build his confidence and openness between you. If he can't get an erection, or only has a partial erection—even when *on his own*—he needs to look at physical causes. He should book a double appointment with his doctor. If he has a woman doctor and feels embarrassed, he may request a male doctor. A double appointment will allow for more time to explore what can be a sensitive issue. Please remember—doctors have heard this problem a thousand times. If he's not happy with his doctor's response he should go to another one. There's no reason why he shouldn't get good advice. Also, visit www.urologychannel.com. In the meantime, you two should engage in affectionate/sensual touching and discuss whether he should simply pleasure you. You should not try to "make him" get an erection.

Women's Sexual Problems

Aside from lacking sexual confidence or not being able to talk about sex, women may experience a number of sexual difficulties. A recent study found that 43 percent of women "lacked sexual interest"—however, this is open to interpretation. Debate has ensued about whether the high result is down to certain issues such as lifestyle choices (for instance, overworking), psychological problems (such as depression) and relationship difficulties (constant arguing will turn you off even the hottest "make-up sex'). Many people are also skeptical about drug companies wanting to cash in on Female Sexual Dysfunction or FSD (the blanket term) by choosing to "medicalize" it rather than looking at it holistically.

Problems that could have an emotional or physical (or combined) basis include:

Vaginismus   Painful spasms of the vaginal muscles before or during intercourse.

Dyspareunia   Pain before, during or after intercourse that many view as distinct from vaginismus. It can be located in different parts of the genitals and is accompanied by varying symptoms, such as vaginal dryness.

Desire problems   No longer feeling sexual desire.

Female Sexual Arousal Disorder (FSAD)   When a woman feels desire but can't get physically aroused for sex.

Anorgasmia or Female Orgasmic Disorder   A woman's inability to achieve orgasm, even with adequate stimulation. There are a variety of causes, whether anatomical, medical, emotional or concerning relationships.

Testosterone   Low levels of testosterone or other hormonal imbalances can lower a woman's sex drive.

For professional advice, speak to your primary care physician for a referral or contact the American Psychotherapy Association (www.americanpsychotherapy.com).

Lack of Desire for Sex

There are many reasons why women end up lacking sexual desire. Up to 40 percent of women complain of lack of desire at some point.

"Too tired for sex"   This is a frequent complaint! I ask a woman to assess her lifestyle. Very often we find she loves her partner and essentially there's no problem in the relationship. However, she simply doesn't have time to look after herself so that she's rested enough to want sex. The choice is to prioritize your relationship, so that you're up for sex on a reasonable basis, or to carry on the way you are—and risk damaging his feelings toward you.

Hormonal changes   These can affect women at different stages of life: during pregnancy and after birth, during peri-menopausal and menopausal changes, as well as during monthly cycle changes. If you think that a lack of desire may be due to hormonal changes you should take a trip to the doctor so your hormones can be checked out. If this *is* found to be the cause, your doctor will advise you of available treatments.

Unhappiness in the relationship There's nothing less sexy than having lots of arguments, giving the "silent treatment" and having general negative feelings in a relationship. Why would you want to sleep with someone you feel you loathe? Sort out the issues causing your relationship stress and you'll find your sex drive returns.

Side effect of medication Medications you're on, such as some antidepressants, can affect your sex drive adversely. Check this out with your doctor and see if there are alternatives you can take.

Sex Addiction

Some debate the existence of "sex addiction." However, I believe that it can exist, like any other addiction. Often sufferers have multiple or cross addictions involving alcohol or drugs. Sometimes sex addiction seems to creep up on an individual. Women, for example, may have taken a few of life's knocks and so choose inappropriate or out-of-character sexual encounters. They then feel badly and go out and try to affirm their self-worth by finding another man so that they can feel desirable. This backfires—he doesn't call—and again they feel bad. It's a vicious circle that keeps reconfirming their lack of self-worth. Some women start to feel, "This is all I deserve." Other women sleep with men right from the start of the relationship, before any trust has been built, and so set a pattern for life. Some signs to look for:

- Do you seek thrills and risks in your sexual relationships?

- Do you jump from one bed to another?

- Do you choose "bad boys"—men who only want one thing?

- Do you feel worthless, empty or dirty after sexual encounters—even when you felt excited at first?

- Are your sexual encounters jeopardizing a relationship, friendships or work in any way?

- Do you go out saying you won't pick up a one-night stand but break that promise to yourself?

- Do you take risks with your sexual health—like "forgetting" to use condoms and/or birth control?

If you recognize yourself in these questions, you need help. Let friends/family know you are making bad choices. Get professional help. For more information call Sex Addicts Anonymous (800-477-8191).

Keeping Your Passion Alive

There are many reasons why couples feel disappointed with sex—usually the culprit is that they've *taken it for granted*. Unlike a car/house that is regularly "serviced/maintained" they treat sex as something that *should just go well*—rather than needing love, care and attention. Other factors, like psychological and mental problems, can affect your desire. If you're depressed or anxious, sexual desire will decline. Lifestyle choices such as smoking, drinking and working long hours will also have a deleterious effect. Arguing and other emotional issues mean emotions in the bedroom cool off. Medical problems and the side effect of some medications can diminish desire. So nurture your relationship and selves and your sex life won't suffer! Here are a few other tips:

Crazy little things   Never forget that the best things come in small packages—and that includes ideas. For example, try "flashlight fun"—using a torch to explore your lover's body under the covers. Or get artistic and buy body-sculpting plaster to make rude sculptures! Have fun directing your own video porn flicks—just don't lose the tapes! Buy fun, sexy surprises—there are all sorts of sex games on the market.

Outside help   See an expert if things are really bad—try the American Association of Sex Educators, Counselors and Therapists (www.aasect.org) to seek a sex therapist.

Medication   Your doctor may be able to prescribe a medication to suit you or your partner, such as testosterone patches, gels or tablets, or other hormone treatments, and pills such as Uprima, Cialis, Viagra or Levitra.

...And Talk to Him in the Morning

So Do You Want a Relationship or a Security Blanket?

The majority of women I meet say they're looking for someone *special*. They want to find a soul mate who'll make them "feel complete." Someone they can hold on to at night, and be there when they "need them." Sounds kind of like a security blanket! Men are not mystical creatures who will turn your life around, make you feel good about yourself, give you constant assurance that your butt doesn't look big (*more on that later!*), and be a lover, friend and confidant at the same time.

This need for "*a man who . . .*" is about our relationship expectations. Where do these come from? For starters, we've all grown up on a diet of fairy tales that our "prince" will rescue us. Second, women's magazines and the media in general, have a lot to answer for—telling us we can expect it all from relationships. A man who can't understand and support us is not worthy of us. Can *you* understand everything about the men you date? No!

Are *you* totally supportive—as well as being a complete love goddess and more? No! So this is the moment of truth, what do you expect? Be honest with yourself and write out your expectations here:

_____

_____

_____

_____

_____

_____

(For example, "I think a man should be willing to try to understand *every* part of me." I actually had a woman say this to me in a life-coaching session recently!) Some expectations are necessary—for example, expecting a man to respect you and not cheat. Never let go of these!

Your Romantic Checklist

Now for fine-tuning. Unfortunately, just as if we're shopping for groceries, women walk around with a romantic checklist in their heads detailing what a man must—and must not—have. After my divorce, my own checklist included, "He must have children." Why? Because I thought a man with children from a previous relationship would understand the needs of my own children. Whom did I marry? A wonderful man without children who's been an amazing stepfather. It takes a special man to do that and I met a special man.

You may not realize you've got a checklist operating in your subconscious. But you may still be guilty of ticking men *off* before they've had a chance to show their worthy qualities. Checklists put a stop to things before a man is given a chance. At different times you'll have different checklists. If you're feeling ready to nest, your checklist may include a man you can "take to meet your parents." If you've just come out of a long-term relationship with a control freak it may include, "He has to be totally relaxed." Typical things on the A to Z of romantic checklists include: he must have the "right" sort of job. Isn't it better that he's a happy gardener than a stressed banker who puts moneymaking before you? Or "he must be at least 5 ft 10 in." So the most fantastic man in the world won't get a look in if he's 5 ft 8 in. If you can dare to dump your checklist, you'll meet a far wider range of men—more to choose from!

Love at First Sight

Some women believe in the love-myth that you'll know immediately if it's "*love*." No! You'll know immediately if it's *lust*! That buzzing, exciting feeling you get when you meet someone new consists of two main things: *1.* Your body chemistry has been excited by theirs; *2.* Your subconscious mind has been sending and receiving all sorts of info about you to each other.

First, science has revealed how our body chemistry reacts when we meet someone we like. We all have special molecules known as major-histo-compatibility-complex (MHC) proteins that help the immune system identify the body's own cells. They mark us out as unique individuals. Nature knows that a couple are more likely to have a healthy baby if certain of their genes are as different as possible. And we're genetically programmed to hunt out these differences. We are helped by the fact that, almost imperceptibly, men with different MHCs *smell* different too. We subconsciously detect this faint odor and, science has shown, we prefer MHCs that are very different from our own. It's appealing to our inner "lust" to reproduce!

Your subconscious works on the social level. What you've been used to as a child growing up—your family patterns of behavior and relationships—you're very good at picking up when someone gives off body language you feel "comfortable" with. That said, we make these decisions very quickly—it's a form of instant gratification. We're sent down the path of finding out more about a man by dating him because we've responded to them in the heat of those initial moments.

There's Only One True Love Out There for Me

I'm not sure where this love-myth started—maybe ancient black and white movies where the heroine, against all odds, would get her guy in the end. The message being, "There's only one true love out there for everyone." Let's get rid of this negative thinking—quickly!

Think about this—you probably *love* many different friends and family members. And, unless you're only just starting to date, you've probably felt *in love* with a number of men. There are loads of singles out there you could potentially share love with. The problem with believing there is "only one" man for you is that if you've had *and lost* a past love (and maybe it left you brokenhearted or finished due to circumstances at the time) you may think it'll never happen again. Many women are so hung up on the "fact" that there can *never* be another, they cast themselves in this role. They give out the vibe that it's "not going to happen for them" and—funnily enough—it doesn't.

We forget that men have intuition too. They're very good at reading women who are lost in "fairy tales"—for example, that they're on a quest for the perfect man or they've loved and lost and there'll never be another. From my own experience, I know this isn't true. In the early days of my first marriage, I was deeply in love with my then husband. We had two beautiful children and I hoped we could work out our differences. I've loved since and, of course, now love my second husband. We have enormous capacity to love—so be positive!

Making Opportunities and Taking Opportunities

We've all regretted not seizing the moment: "Why didn't I just kiss him when I had the chance?" If you think failure to seize moments causes regret in dating, then not taking opportunities causes even more. Think of "moments" as things that *enrich* your life and "opportunities" as things that *change* your life. They're both potentially great, but opportunities are simply on a bigger scale. We've all heard friends say, "I could have asked that great guy out, but I didn't have the confidence, courage, guts, etc. to do it."

Key strategies you can use to increase your dating opportunities:

1. Be aware of your surroundings when you're out—tune in to what's going on rather than tuning it out. If you spot a gorgeous new guy at your gym, think about how to say hello. Paying attention doesn't just help you meet men—it also helps with every aspect of your relationship once you're

114

in one. If you can spot the opportunity to meet the absolutely stunning man you've noticed in the offices next door, then once you're dating him you can also spot opportunities to deepen your intimacy, to surprise him and keep things fresh!

2. Don't just wait for opportunities to arise: make opportunities for yourself. Successful daters arm themselves with knowledge they use to increase their chances of making and taking opportunities. Such people never stop learning about what's going on socially: they always know about upcoming singles events, and they listen when they hear six new recruits are joining the office.

3. Enlist your friends. Women who make and take opportunities are willing to share their knowledge. They tell each other about social events, go out to clubs together, and maximize their opportunities. They can see "two heads are..."

Finally, spotting that opportunity to meet someone new or develop depth to your relationship will become part of your life skills. You'll see things coming and have the courage to take them on. Your homework: this month spot a dating or romantic opportunity and go for it!

Are You Guilty of Problem Behavior?

There are four general types of behavior profiles that cause problems for relationships, making them hard work and shortening their "shelf-life." I call these "Problem behaviors" or "P behaviors."

Prima Donna   Self-centered and demanding with no empathy for others' situations—including boyfriends. You feel no one understands you. *Effect on relationships:* If he doesn't worship you, you get icy and huffy. *Change:* For every demand you make, give in to one of his.

People Pleaser   The "yes" person and perennial doormat who'll go along with anything. She fears standing up for herself—worries that no one will like the real her. *Effect on relationships:* A man might get tired of a woman with no "mind of her own" or he may take advantage of her willing nature. *Change:* At least once daily, speak your mind. Also, when he asks what *you* want to do on a date, choose something—don't say "whatever you want."

Passion Victim   Your friends can count on you for dramatics. Unlike the Prima Donna, your dramatics revolve around their lives as much as yours. You'll make a mountain out of any molehill. *Effect on relationships:* He'll find you hard work. At first curious about your dramatics, he'll tire of them over time. *Change:* Calm down and enjoy letting little things roll off your back.

Perfectionist   Everything must be perfect and your definition of perfect is yours. This means you're a control freak who wants things done your way. *Effect on relationships:* He can never be right. You can never share doing things. He'll feel intimidated. *Change:* Each day, practice doing something differently—try others' suggestions.

See "Do You Say Yes When You Want to Say No?" on page 118.

Do You Say Yes
When You Want to Say No?

Learning to assert yourself is a valuable tool for your relationship and any aspect of life. Whether you find it impossible to say no to the new guy who pressures you into sex, or say yes to everything he suggests even when it's the last thing you'd choose to do on a date, asserting yourself is an important skill. Any such circumstance will cause less worry if you know you'll speak your mind. Women who aren't assertive worry men won't like them if they set limits—but believe me, men respect you *more* if you do!

1. Know and stick to your limits. If you don't want to have sex with him until you're sure of your feelings—and his—explain this to him early on.

2. Believe your judgement. You're right—the man who keeps trying to cajole you into sex or anything else needs to be shown where you stand. This doesn't make you a bad person.

3. Give yourself permission to say no. This doesn't mean you leave behind being a "yes person" who seizes opportunities, but you can't say yes to everything! If you're dating a man with lazy-guy syndrome who leaves all the arrangements to you, and you've organized the last four dates and don't have time this week—ask him to do it!

4. Whenever you discuss a problem in your relationship, treat it like taking back faulty merchandise. Practice what you're going to say, keep calm, and repeat yourself as often as needed to get your message through. You're less likely to be railroaded into backing down.

5. Remember, asserting yourself is not being aggressive—you shouldn't have to raise your voice when learning to say no to him.

How to Flirt

Flirting makes us feel good. A recent survey found that nearly 50 percent of men had "flirted" in the last week, while only 37 percent of women had. So, guys are doing it more! Research from the Social Issues Research Centre in the UK found that women use flirting to sort out their level of interest in a "Mr. Possibility." This is why men get confused—she's flirting but then she says "No" to a date. It's not uncommon for men to use a form of "courtesy flirting" to make a woman feel good, even though they have no intention of asking her out.

Flirting is *not* teasing! Flirting involves subtle signs of interest while teasing suggests "action" is on the cards when it's not. Some flirting "Dos":

- Giving knowing looks is a starting point—they say, "I find you attractive."

- The eyes are the windows to the soul, so ensure you've got a glint in yours.

- Give compliments, but only if you mean them. Men love compliments as much as we do.

- Be flirty with the things you say, making them sound slightly mischievous.

- If you've given him your number and he uses it, keep the conversation light, fun and *short* so he wants more!

- Be playful. During a goodnight kiss you can tickle him with your fingertips. A little flirty laughter goes a long way, too.

- Play obvious games. If he asks you out, say you're busy for "two weeks"—watch his face drop and then say, "But I can fit you in on Friday." (Choose a day three days away.)

Where to Meet Men

Something I can't say often enough is *widen your circle of opportunity*. If you've been going to the same singles bar for three months and you haven't met anyone—go somewhere else! If you've been hanging out at the same gym and not struck lucky—choose another gym! You're responsible for choosing new venues, seizing opportunities to chat to that new man at work, and letting acquaintances know you're in the "market." Try speed dating, Internet sites, agencies and the many singles events available in most cities. There are single men out there—no excuses!

Your safety   Use these simple tips to keep safe while not inhibiting your sense of freedom and independence.

- Take his phone number and use caller ID blocking if possible when dialing so that you stay in control of contact.

- Meet in a public place in the daytime—a coffee date is always a great starting point.

- Tell friends or family where you're going. Or even bring a friend, particularly if you've met someone off the Internet—if he objects, it makes you wonder about his motives. Alternatively, get a friend to phone you 45 minutes into your date to check all's well, and use this call as a "get out" if it's not going well.

- Keep your cell on and carry a personal alarm— you should do this anyway.

- Until you know him, do not go to his home or somewhere isolated, even if you feel you trust him at first.

- Finally, if your intuition tells you something's wrong—believe it! We were given this "sixth sense" to warn us of unusual body language— barely visible to the eye but clear to our subconscious.

Get Lucky in Love!

Many believe love is controlled by fate and luck. Yes, certain things you can't control—for example, the weather and the behavior of others. But the rest of life and love and how "lucky" you are is up to you. Call it making your own luck, or simply behaving in ways that enhance your love life—here are some key principles to help you.

Let's turn to some classic sayings to help you get lucky:

1. *If at first you don't succeed, try, try again.*
   Women who are lucky in love keep trying because they know giving up will get them nowhere. I'll use a personal example to illustrate. After my divorce I thought I might never find the right man, but I kept trying. I dated a lot of men—some were duds and some delightful—and then I met the man who became my second husband. So never give up!

2. *You're mistress of your own destiny.* If you leave your love life in the hands of others, you'll never get what you want. But if you take control and get out there, keeping your eyes open, you'll reap many rewards. You make your own "luck" by making your own decisions about who to go out with, when to end something that's not working, and when to take a leap of faith even though you're not sure of a man's potential—give that shy guy a chance and he might turn out to be fantastic!

3. *Every cloud has a silver lining.* When you're lucky in love, you can find something useful even in a "bad" experience when things don't go your way. You know that you may learn something about romance, find a new path, or grow in maturity through facing this "cloud."

Why Men Don't Call

You've had a couple of dates and all seems great. He's got your number now and you're anticipating date number three. But he *never* calls. You get on the phone with your friends and dissect everything. Were there any signs? Did you do something wrong? Has he had a car crash since your last date? The answer to these questions is "No!" You haven't done anything wrong and he isn't in the hospital dying. There are three main reasons why he doesn't call:

1. Simple nerves on his part. He's wondering, "Does she really like me?" In his little mind he decides for some reason you're not as keen as he is—so he doesn't call. He's thought of ten reasons why you might not like him. Yes, men can be that insecure—just ask a male friend.

2. You have to face facts. He decided he didn't like you enough to take it further. Most men will not

do what we'd do in this situation. We'd tell a guy—"I'm just not interested" or "I like you as a friend." They won't! They think it's better ("easier") to just leave things. They don't realize you're going to be tormented by insecurity.

3. Sometimes men lose the impetus. Things get in the way, particularly if he's quite independent or has lots of hobbies. He forgets to call because he's busy. He then feels embarrassed and lets a couple of days go by. Then he decides it's too late anyway.

The message If he doesn't call and you have his number, then call him for a chat and sound out his enthusiasm—or lack of. If you don't have his number or he doesn't seem keen, forget him and move on!

How Men Think

Get inside a man's mind and you'd be amazed—they simply don't think the way we do. If you want to improve your relationships you need to understand this. I like to see differences as good—we complement each other. The ancient Chinese recognized this in their Yin-Yang symbolism. Difference can lead to harmony—if we *understand him* rather than treat him as an alien.

Anthropologists realize our distant ancestors had complex roles. At times, everyone in the "cave group" had to chip in with different tasks. However, as women gave birth and suckled their offspring, their roles essentially developed around the village. They had to "multi-task," meeting the demands of infants, the elderly and tending any animals or plants that were raised by the group.

Men, on the other hand, had to get out in the jungle or on the plain and hunt. They had to focus on bringing down the kill and getting it home—often over long journeys, where pure survival took precedent over any niceties. They were truly goal oriented, with few distractions.

How do these differences affect modern relationships? Evolution is very slow and so genetically we're still programmed to behave in these ways. Men, on the whole, like to keep things straightforward in relationships, as in the rest of their life. They are goal directed and their goal is to get the relationship going and then let it "hum along nicely." Women have a strong desire to nurture things along, question the way things are, and long for deep communication. A man thinks, "The meat's on the table—what's there to talk about?"

Working with the Way Men Think

To improve the relationship with your "ancient man," you need to deal with his goal-oriented thinking. Try these:

- We think differently—so learn from each other. Sometimes every little thing doesn't need analysis. We should try out this element of men's thinking. When you catch yourself wanting to dissect everything about your conversation with your boss—and he's rolling his eyes—drop it. Dissect it with a girlfriend.

- Your type of thinking is not necessarily better than his! At the end of the day, put both thinking styles to good use. If he's got a problem with a female colleague, give him some tips to help him understand her. And vice versa.

- Arguments can start when either one of you refuses to acknowledge that you both may think about things differently—and they're both equally valid.

- It's true—two heads are better than one!

- Think twice before asking him what *he's thinking*. This can be incredibly annoying to a man. You're unlikely to get a straight answer. Tell him your thoughts instead, for example, "I was thinking . . ."

- Don't try to read his mind. A bad habit we women have! You can't—so *ask* him, when you need to.

- Men's thoughts usually go from A to B. Ours go from A to K around to P and finish at Z. You don't have to share all these points with him— he'll tune you out anyway.

- Silence is golden. Men are often quite content with a bit of silence. It's not always negative!

How Men Feel

A typical assumption women make is that because a man may not express his feelings or he has difficulty when he does (think Hugh Grant in *Four Weddings and a Funeral*), he may not feel as deeply as she does. This simply isn't true. Men do feel things deeply but often contain those feelings more than we do and simply believe they're putting themselves on the line, unnecessarily, to express them.

It's important to remember that a man does have feelings, but they may NOT be the same as yours. Just as if you and your best friend were both in love, she may feel different aspects of her relationships are more important than the things you feel strongly about. We're all individuals.

The roots of our differences lie with our distant ancestors again. In our nurturing role, back by the "campfire," we simply had to be in tune with the needs of our newborns. We had to know when their crying was over something basic, like tiredness, or something more important, such as illness. Likewise, ancient men had to learn to suppress feelings, particularly fear, when out hunting and fishing. They needed to concentrate on the task and couldn't be distracted. Feelings came second to the job at hand—quite the opposite of ancient women, for whom feelings were important. Understanding this can go a long way to accepting our differences. A big sign of his feelings comes from his behavior—does he treat you well? Then he's got the right feelings!

Working with the Way Men Feel

Your relationships will be much smoother if you get to grips with some basic rules about his emotions. Try these:

- Men recognize they have feelings for someone new but don't always want to delve too deeply into these. Life is much easier if they don't feel pressured to talk about these new "sensations."

- Often men know they feel something but can't identify it—is it simply sexual excitement or do they really care? They find it harder to label their feelings. We can tell quite quickly if it's *lust*, *like* or *love*.

- Strong feelings can provoke anxiety in men. Sometimes they choose to ignore them—and they may lose out in a relationship. Men may have more sexual partners in their lives but they fall in love less frequently than we do.

- Because they may want to "ignore" strong feelings, they often don't have the relationship vocabulary to describe them. Keep it simple when talking about your new relationship.

- A lifetime of programming *not* to show their feelings won't be changed overnight. Even their moms told them, "Big boys don't cry." Why should they believe any differently? Coax it out of them.

- What you see is what you get. You may have a million wonderful emotions. He may feel only one.

- He may learn to open up with you—but don't drag it out of him in front of his friends!

- Ask what he's thinking and you may get an idea what he's feeling.

- Tell him your feelings in moderate doses.

One-Night Stands

If you're looking for love and a relationship, then you should avoid one-night stands. Only a small percentage of relationships blossom from a one-night stand. Having no-strings sex is absolutely fine if that's all you want (play safe!). However, one-night stands can have a high emotional cost. I've had countless women tell me they thought there was a special connection and so they had sex right away—only to be incredibly disappointed when he didn't call.

Why do so many men do this? Unfortunately, we're living in the REAL world, not the PC (politically correct) IDEAL world where no one is judged. Many men still judge a woman unfairly if she has quick sex. They figure she must be doing it with every other guy. So they're thinking, "I'm not so special am I?" Really, trust me, many men have a fairly low opinion of themselves in this regard.

At the same time they're confident enough to take sex that's easy and simply enjoy it. They're far more capable of having no-emotions sex and enjoying the physical side of a one-night stand. There are men who feel that one-night stands cheapen *them*—however, they're rare. A survey found that 98 percent of single men would take sex that was easy without too many qualms.

So you've been warned. If you want more than sex then don't have sex with him until you know what he wants too. Over time, it'll become fairly obvious whether he sees you as just a casual date or is really interested.

Men and Love

Funnily enough, we're bad at giving men a chance if they haven't leapt straight off our romantic checklist. Men are even worse at this! In some ways they're pickier about whom they fall in love with. Going back to their ancient roots sheds some light on this. Their genes tell them to spread their seed (that is, have lots of sex) but it's quite another thing to look after and provide for those off-spring. So, somewhere in their genetic code they seem to be more wary of settling into a *love-thing*.

Knowing this means you have to be fairly subtle at sliding them into that *love-thing*. The better a man feels around you, the more likely he is to acknowledge deep feelings and fall in love. Of course, some men love a woman who's a challenge. However, most men want to enter a comfort zone that's probably reminiscent of how their mother nurtured them—but they'd never admit this!

So, the keys to engendering a good feeling around you are:

- Make things easy. Know what you'd like to do without being bossy.

- Be affectionate—but not in front of his friends, if that irritates him.

- Ensure you're not waiting for his call—but enjoy him when you're together.

- Laugh at his jokes! It's simple—men feel good when they think they entertain you.

- Show you care, but without seeming desperate.

- Once you've got this good-vibe going, he's more likely to start acknowledging strong feelings about you.

Men and Commitment

Even if a man falls in love it may still be an issue for him to *commit*. The "C" word holds all sorts of "darker" meanings for him. Many men see it as a loss of freedom, sexual adventure and even youth. Being in love doesn't necessarily mean "forever," but to commit—either to marriage or living together—well, this sends all sorts of alarm bells ringing. So, just as getting him to fall in love means providing him with a fun, inviting comfort zone, you need to be aware that getting him to the next hurdle also involves making sure it feels good for him.

Getting a man to the point of commitment is full of hurdles. One of their worst fears is that they might actually get so comfortable in this *love-thing* that'll they go from being, say, a *25-year-old guy-about-town* straight to a *middle-aged type*. That's scary!

The most interesting thing about men reaching their "commitment threshold" (as I call it) is that it takes them longer to get there but—once there—they're less likely to dump the relationship than a woman. Women seek 70 percent of divorces. Men, on the other hand, think, "It's working OK, why go through the torment again of getting to know someone else?" Remember, commitment makes them vulnerable—so be gentle! Be confident—his thinking will catch up with yours, just give him time. Watch out for the signs that show he's ready—he'll open up to you verbally with time.

The Green-eyed Monster

Jealousy is a problem that most of us run into at some point. Recent research has shown that we have a "jealous gene." This probably served some sort of adaptive purpose in the relationships of ancient men and women. Feeling jealous was probably protective of the family unit and so sustained family groups against the odds when life was difficult.

We are not ancient women, though, and so need to rise above destructive jealousy. To start with, acknowledge any jealous feelings—they're OK. You're not superhuman. You may have them when some gorgeous girl gives your man the "eye" or if he spends too much time with his friends. It's *how* you respond to them, and *what* you do with them, that counts. So, what should you do?

1. Identify what it is that actually makes you feel jealous in this situation. Is it that you're feeling

"ugly"—rather than the fact that he responded to another woman giving him a "look"?

2. Once identified—sort it. In the example above, do something about the way you believe you look. If you two have gone out for drinks and you're wearing old sweats and haven't washed your hair, you'll feel jealous of every passing woman with shiny locks.

3. Substitute a positive thought for your jealous thought. For example, "I'm a fantastic person so what am I worried about?" Repetition works!

4. Tell your partner you're having an "iffy" moment so that he knows you're trying to get over any jealousy issues. Hopefully, he'll be supportive.

Sexual Jealousy

Here are some *Golden Rules* on sexual jealousy:

- Past lovers are NEVER any good! Never start chatting about what your ex was like in bed unless you're saying how selfish and bad he was! If you beat around the bush and sound at all ambiguous, it's easy for your lover to misinterpret what you're saying and feel sexual jealousy. Anyway, why bring up an ex-lover?

- Beware of flirting when you're out together. When it comes to being "territorial," men and women are just as bad as each other. For every story you've heard about a man getting possessive in public when he thinks his partner's being flirted with, there's another one of a woman getting jealous. We feel threatened when someone is interested in our mate. So it's best to learn how to deal with feelings of sexual jealousy.

- There'll always be good-looking men and women wherever you go. You both have to deal with this. Don't get involved when someone tries to chat you up. If either you or your lover gets a buzz from being chatted up, look deeper into this need. It's about reassurance for yourself. Be firm with yourself and don't get into tricky situations that upset your partner. Find things that boost your ego and don't involve flirting.

- And if your partner is jealous without reason— don't pander to it! If he calls ten times a day asking what you're "up to" cut the conversation short or change it to something constructive. He's got to control this tendency, so set your boundaries.

Actions Speak Louder Than Words

A really clued-in woman knows that a man's behavior speaks louder than words. We all love Hugh Grant in his mumbling, bumbling, *difficult-to-express-himself-type* film roles. But we tend to hate the real thing! If you're with a man who finds communication difficult, watch for the gestures that say he cares. They include:

- Giving you a pet nickname.

- Arranging a surprise meal or cooking for you.

- Giving you a surprise gift.

- Showing some sort of public affection—even if it's only a gentle touch to your back.

- Sending you jokey texts, e-mails—it shows he wants to make you smile.

- Calling for no apparent reason—it means he wants to hear your voice.

- Opening up about problems at work.

- Introducing you as his girlfriend.

- Offering to help with something at your home.

Signs that he's not serious include:

- Giving his friends more attention than you.

- Saying, "Let's take our time."

- Saying he's not sure what he's looking for.

- You do most of the phone calling and "chasing."

- Never taking the initiative about what to do/where to go.

- Never talking to you about anything important— such as work, family.

- Making no effort to tidy his place when you come over—although he may simply be a slob!

- If you have a "gut feeling" that his heart's not in it—listen to your intuition.

Retaining Mystery Is Different from Playing Games!

In these days of wearing our hearts on our sleeves, it's easy to forget that effusiveness about personal and intimate matters can be very threatening. Retaining mystery is different from playing games—those can put a man off. I like to think of it as revealing yourself slowly—like a sensual strip tease. What's sexier? Ripping your clothes off and lunging at someone while naked? Or slowly and seductively stripping away a layer at a time? It's the same with personal information—slowly does it—then he'll want to know even more! Here are some simple strategies to keep him interested until he's in love:

- Avoid the "L" words—"love" or "like"—until he's really comfortable with you.

- Don't let him know you're having, for example, mood swings over work.

148

- Don't go on about past crises, such as telling him every detail about your parents' horrible divorce.

- If he's got plans, so have you! Even if those plans are to do a face mask.

- When he phones, give him five minutes. Don't let him think you've got all the time in the world.

- When people call your cell, don't tell him who's just called you.

- Space your dates at first. Twice a week for the first three weeks is plenty. Don't tell him what you're doing when you're not seeing him. He's not your keeper.

- Don't let him know that it took you an hour to get ready. Your personal habits are private!

- Don't discuss illness in detail unless it's something very obvious.

The Art of Conversation with Men

Women have become so competitive that men now say they feel that they're in a competition when on a date! It's great that you're top dog at work, or a black belt in karate. But with a man you should be an equal—not a rival. Remember, men tend to have a "need-to-know" style of communication—they may not want to tell you every little thing—so slowly, slowly! Try the following for cool, not competitive, conversation when first dating:

- Avoid the "bulldog" phenomenon—if you disagree on a topic, let it go. Don't wrestle with it like a bone.

- Don't use your "intuition" to always be right, saying, "I know this because my intuition tells me." That's the easy way out when you don't have facts to back your point.

- Avoid the "broken record syndrome" where you repeat things. Research has found that women repeat themselves more often than men.

- Don't use "verbal slaps" when you don't agree—such as telling a man he's "silly" or "doesn't understand." Men take these things deeply.

- Great conversation is like a *gentle* game of tennis—not a hard-fought tournament.

- Never use "shut-down" lines that stop conversation dead, such as, "You wouldn't understand—you're a man!"

- Variety is the spice of good conversation, so cover lots of topics.

- Ask him what *he* knows about a topic. This is like giving him a "stroke," generating love vibes.

- Watch your vocal tone. If you're warm, soft and sensual you're more likely to be listened to—not shrill and demanding!

Have a Life

There's nothing sadder than a woman sitting by the phone waiting for a man to call, or checking her cell for messages every couple of minutes. Have you ever checked a line because you thought it might be malfunctioning? Most have, but this is really unhealthy for a relationship. Would you like to go out with a man who waited for you, like a doormat with no life?

I call this the "Princess Syndrome" as, once upon a time (in the Middle Ages), princesses waited for their knights to charge by. Why do you think men would find the Princess Syndrome attractive? They don't. Word of warning here—a man who wants to control you will expect you to wait for his call. That's not healthy! Here are some tips to break the Princess habit:

- Force yourself not to answer the phone one evening per week. Be busy doing what you want. Period!

- Put a fun message on your answering machine. Not one that lists every possible place you might be found—that sounds like you're obsessive and overly keen to be found!

- Ask a friend to be your "crisis buddy"—when you feel like calling the new man in your call her instead.

- Do not make crank calls at any time—ever!

- Do NOT drop plans you've made if he calls wanting to see you.

- Make the other things you have to do interesting—so you really want to do them and aren't grudgingly "keeping busy" because you know you should.

Dating and Your Friends

We have a terrible habit of dumping our girlfriends when we fall for someone new. This is something many women regret, especially when the guy's gone and her ex-best girlfriend doesn't really want to know. So you need to ensure you don't neglect your girlfriends when you fall in love. Try these:

- Make dates with her too—and stick to them.

- Keep any long-term plans you've made with her—like that long-awaited trip to Australia. The new man will just have to wait.

- Every time you text message your new love, text message her too.

- Try to get him to bring a friend along for a double date. Nothing serious, just four people getting together to have fun.

- If she already has a boyfriend, make up a double date with him.

- Never forget you can have both—a relationship and a best friend.

The other big problem—from the opposite direction—is *envy*. Sometimes you might find that your friends envy *you*, especially if they're not in love, or think you *always* get the guy, or maybe they liked him, too. How to prevent envy:

- Let her know how much you value her friendship.

- Talk to her about your worry that she's not happy with your new relationship. Hiding these thoughts makes them fester.

- Don't drone on about how wonderful Mr. Possibility is—make sure your conversation revolves around things besides him.

- At the end of the day, if she has a big problem with envy—she'll have to change!

The Rule of Three

There are three hurdles that the vast majority of couples face—I call them the *Rule of Three*—and they can make or break a new relationship. Let's go through them, so you know how they work:

Third Date If you make it past the first date then, by the third date, you'll probably have decided whether there is real interest *or not*. It's usually after the third date that women complain he didn't call. By the fourth date, they find they really start "getting to know him" since they've made it that far. By the third date you can see past your initial chemistry a bit and not have your judgment clouded by it. So treat date No. 3 like the first—be on your best behavior if you really like him.

Three Weeks Having made it to three weeks, this is when people start dropping their guard. You may suddenly find they have an irritating habit they've kept hidden. Or else something you thought was "sexy" actually turns you off—such as his laugh! This is the point at which one or the other of you may back off, as little things take on a bigger meaning.

Three Months   This is a critical time for "big decisions" to pop up—and make waves in any relationship that isn't solid. You may want to hear that he "loves you" because you feel that way. You may find that one of you is always spending nights at the other's home—so topics like "moving in" come up. How well you discuss these things will determine whether you fall at this important hurdle.

Does My Butt Look Too Big?

There are some things we can't resist asking a man—even if we *know* we'll never get straight answers. Men find it really hard to walk that line between honesty and tact. They hate the idea of hurting a girlfriend over such questions but worry they'll be caught lying. So give them a break! Think about it. The question, "Does my butt look big in this?" is tantamount to him asking you, "Does my penis look small?" How would you feel put on the spot with that question? It's really more about your esteem than your size! Men know we fret about our body size, so you'll really make him squirm. Here are some other questions that men find hard to answer and so you should *avoid*—or at least not ask them *directly*:

- Do you like my friends? You can ask this one only after a few months together.

- Do you like my mother? *Never* ask this one! Let this relationship develop slowly.

- Do you love me? *Never* ask this one—wait and see if he tells you at some point after the six-month mark. Before that and you're very lucky! Some men never can say those three little words—so do their actions say it for them?

- When did you *know* you loved me? Unless he's the rare soppy type, he won't be able to answer this. Men fall in love but can rarely identify when they knew. Unlike *us*—we can tell them the minute and second when *we* knew!

- Was your ex more attractive, sexier, funnier, more popular, than me? Don't even go there! He's with you now.

Bad Hair Days and Intimacy

Many of us may not fall prey to serious problems like clinical depression or eating disorders, but we all have "bad hair days" when we feel ugly inside and out! Part of the ability to achieve true intimacy with a lover is to be able to *admit* when you're having a bad hair day. Most of us are comfortable confiding to friends, but too many women worry they'll be rejected or ignored by romantic partners if they own up to feeling bad about themselves. Confiding negative feelings is an important part of intimacy, though—and bad hair days are the very days that we most need a hug! Try these methods for improving intimacy with him:

1. Choose your moment. When you tell him how you're feeling, you want him to be ready to listen. If he's in a bad mood or stressed out from work, he may not be receptive to your feelings—intimacy is a two-way street.

2. Reveal your feelings gradually. Deeper intimacy comes through revealing yourself step by step. It's like peeling an onion: slowly, layer after layer, you get to the core. The man you're relating to hopefully feels trust building between you and starts to reveal his feelings step by step too. But if you flood him with *everything* that's in your heart and soul all at once, he may back off.

3. When letting a man in, tell him why you've chosen to talk to him about this—because you trust him and feel close already, or you want to feel even closer. At intimate moments like these, remind your partner how much he means to you.

4. Don't let fear of rejection stop you from reaching out when you're feeling bad.

5. Be good to *yourself* on bad hair days—relax, nap, see a movie, and ask him for a hug!

Your Intuition Radar

We were given a "sixth sense," our intuition, for good reason—to sense danger back when we lived on the plain and in the jungle. *Real* dangers were around every corner and our ancestors paid attention to the feeling of hairs rising on the back of their necks. However, I find women today simply don't want to pay attention to their intuition.

What sorts of things does your "intuition" tell you? Your intuition is like your subconscious policewoman. If you're about to call the man you just met but you have this niggling "suspicion" that you might sound desperate—listen to this suspicion. Your intuition has picked up all sorts of information about him at a subconscious level. Like a radar searching for "signals," it has, for example, detected that this new guy is reserved. So calling may frighten him off. We may choose to consciously ignore such signals but our intuition is a clever piece of our make-up trying to alert us to situations. Here are some more things our intuition radar tells us:

- The outfit we've chosen might just be a little over the top, so dress it down a notch.

- We're "gushing" too much information about ourselves in our conversation. Tone it down and ask about him.

- We don't think he really likes us. Your radar's probably noticed him eye-up other women who've walked into the bar.

- Finally, our butt *does* look big in this new outfit we made a rushed decision about—believe it, it may do.

- He's unreliable. Many women choose to ignore it when their intuition says this!

Your Dating Confidence

The more confident you are, the more successful your relationships! Research shows similar levels of confidence attract each other. If you lack confidence you'll subconsciously choose a man who also lacks confidence. His lack of confidence may come out in toxic ways, like: *1.* Bullying you; *2.* Two-timing you to build his own self-worth; *3.* He may lie, cheat and undermine you—because he knows your confidence is too low to stand up for yourself; *4.* He may simply be like you—and the two of you together forge a relationship where you both fret and worry about things, or get into a rut, and don't have the confidence to try new ways of relating or improving things. Here are the "dirty dozen" signs that tell a man that a woman feels unworthy:

1. Shy and awkward body language.

2. Not saying what she wants to do on a date.

3. Picking at food—fear of eating in public.

4. Appearing eager to please.

5. Feigning interest in something—when clearly she's not.

6. Wanting to know every detail of his relationship history—she doesn't have confidence in the fledgling relationship.

7. Asking to be compared to an ex.

8. Gushing about her romantic successes—she's got something to prove.

9. Bragging about how many men are after her *now*.

10. Claiming she's not looking for anything right now. ("The lady doth protest too much!")

11. Being overly flirtatious to prove she's a sex kitten.

12. Asking overly personal information about him. She's lost control of her tongue!

Building Your Dating Confidence Will Improve Your Relationships

It's vitally important to build your general dating confidence so that you meet the most worthy men and have positive relationships. You can choose to continue to run yourself down, expect little from men and generally continue along a negative path. Or you can choose to raise that dating confidence.

Try these:

- To practice saying what *you'd* like to do with him, try saying what you'd like to do with friends and colleagues.

- Many women judge their "date-ability" by their size. If they're large they think they have nothing to offer. You can choose to focus on your size or you can choose three attributes you have to focus on.

- Stop trying to please men. Men love strong women so say things you mean, express your opinions and views.

- Don't allow bad past experiences to cloud your dating *now*. Select one good date from the past and remind yourself of this one.

- Seize dating opportunities. If the nice man in the elevator at work suggests coffee—say "Yes." Even if you don't like him, it's good dating practice.

- Set goals, if, for example, you like someone at your gym. *Goal 1*—go and exercise next to him. *Goal 2*—smile at him. *Goal 3*—ask how to use a piece of equipment, and so on.

- Practice flirting by flirting with your local shopkeeper or the salesmen in a department store. Smile nicely, throw your head back, laugh and enjoy your interaction with them!

Getting Off on the Right Foot for a Relationship

Let's say things are feeling good. You've passed the second "rule of three"—being together for more than three weeks. Here are some golden rules for building a relationship out of dating:

- Expect to have good fun and it might become a romance. Expect a romance and it's less likely to happen.

- Keep things in balance. If it feels like love it might be—but ensure you keep the rest of your life going so that you're not left high and dry after a month together. He dumps you—you're friends are angry, as you've ignored them, and you're behind at work, having spent four weeks daydreaming about him and his babies.

- Possessiveness is an ugly trait. The more you cultivate "caring independence," the happier you'll be in each other's company.

- A great saying to remember when you're dating is: "You attract bees with honey—not vinegar!"

- Both self-respect and respect for him are critical to developing a satisfying relationship. He's a unique human being—as you are. Respect his feelings, wishes and points of view—as you expect him to respect yours.

- A big mistake is trying to *change* him. If he's got faults you *hate*—he's probably not right in the long run. If they're little nit-picky things, with time he can change those. You can change *yours* (yes, you'll have irritating habits too!) and accept the rest.

- Personal responsibility is critical to your developing love. You're responsible for your behavior. He doesn't *make* you behave a certain way. You have choices, so make wise ones!

Married Men Myths

I'd be rich if I'd had $1 for every time I've been told a woman knows her married (or otherwise taken) partner is going to be all hers one day—and then it doesn't happen! Check out the figures: about 42 percent of attached men admit to being unfaithful at some point. Only about 1 percent of these ever leaves his partner. Not good odds!

Why women get involved with married men Usually they have low self-esteem and feel they only deserve "crumbs." It can be more complex—they might thrive on risk, excitement and hot sex. They may genuinely not want a full relationship—if so, why not have a part-time one with a single guy? Real intimacy frightens them and so their married guy will never be a threat. But love with a married man is not a game.

Why you can't trust a married man They're usually after sex and excitement, period! They don't want another relationship—they have that! What they don't have is excitement. You provide that—if you're stupid enough.

What to do Tell him it's over and give yourself breathing space. Do not be conned into letting him come over to talk about it. Get a crisis buddy—a girlfriend you can call at times when you feel weak. Tell your mom—she'll talk sense into you. Don't take his calls. Look around the single scene—get out and find someone who can have a relationship—or just "fun," if that's all you want!

Coping with Infidelity

In an ideal world infidelity wouldn't happen. But it does and it's all too common. It's a myth that relationships can't survive it. Some simply survive it better than others. Here are the things to consider and try if one of you is unfaithful:

- Do you both want to work it out? If the answer's "no" there's little hope.

- Don't make rash decisions in the immediate aftermath of discovery.

- If you're both committed to working it out, take a long look at why the person had the affair. There are so many reasons, such as stupidity, anger, revenge, feeling neglected, not thinking, sex, power.

- This is a time for honesty—otherwise it won't work. You've had the pain. Now you need to face the truths.

- Facing the truth does not mean having to reveal every last detail of the affair. Let the person who has been cheated on choose how much detail they want. But remember, once you've asked for detail you can't go back. There may be hurtful things in the detail. Think before you ask.

- Expect a variety of emotions—just like a bereavement. You've lost trust—this is tough, and you'll range through anger, despair, bitterness and utter disbelief.

- Do not keep throwing up the affair in every little argument you have. This is very destructive and tells the partner who's been unfaithful that you'll never forget. This gives you less of a chance to work things out.

Meeting Each Other's Families

When you take on him you take on his family (and friends!) too. You'd be naive to think otherwise. Unless he's an orphan, you'll have to share him sometimes—as he'll have to share you. Here are some tips for playing happy families:

- Treat his mother like a rival and she'll become one. It's a self-fulfilling prophecy. Instead, encourage him to have a good relationship with her.

- You love him and she raised him so show her respect.

- If he has an interfering mother—for example, one who wants to make his decisions for him—talk about it with him. Present a united but caring front to her and she'll have her wings clipped.

- Never ridicule his family—leave that to him, if he wants to.

- That said, families can be strange. You don't have to spend time with his family if they're difficult or abusive. Let him know why you're making other plans when he goes there for the weekend.

- Agree how much time you'll spend with both your families and divide this in two so that each gets equal time.

- Alternate spending special occasions at each other's homes.

- Try to stay out of family arguments. They happen but you should ignore them.

- Give him a list of his family birthdays so he can send out cards for his side and you can for your side. Nothing's more irritating than becoming the "diary secretary" for both families—unless you like those jobs!

- All these rules apply to his family—and yours.

Energize Your Love Life!

Many women complain of a lack of sizzle and spontaneity in their love life. Slipping into a routine with a partner can lead to boredom. If you find yourself never having enough time, that can also cause your love life to lose steam. Here are a few simple things that can recharge your love life:

1. Sex! Oxytocin, the hormone released during orgasm, makes you feel sleepy at first—but then you're reinvigorated. Research shows that having sex twice a week keeps people looking and feeling younger. Use it or lose it! So keep the chemistry alive between you.

2. Exercise! Exercise *gives* energy. Only TOO much exercise is detrimental. Make sure you and your partner get moderate exercise consisting of three 30-minute aerobic sessions per week plus 20

minutes daily of something like a vigorous walk together. Keeping fit together can be another way of bonding.

3. Flexibility! Keeping an open and flexible attitude toward life will keep your relationship alive. Habits and routine are fine, but they kill romance if relied on all the time.

4. Good food! Ensuring you're both in tip top shape will help your relationship, because you'll have the energy you need to invest in it. What you eat determines to a large extent how energetic you feel. Food is fuel! A diet of pre-packed foods high in sugar and fat won't fuel your busy life. Make sure you eat fresh fruit and vegetables daily. Drink water or fruit juices instead of soda. Avoid fried foods that leave you lethargic. Eat slow-burning carbohydrates (pasta, whole-wheat bread) for energy.

5. Fun! Do something childish together. Swing on swings, fly a kite, watch your favorite kids' movie (*The Sound of Music*?)—these help you find your inner child. And children have energy!

Keeping Romance Alive

Couples forget that the *only things* separating their relationship from simply being a strong friendship is romance and sex. Romance makes what you have that much more special. Like flirting, romance tells your lover that you want to *make him feel fantastic*. In a loving relationship romance is not forgotten. Try these:

- Create a love-tape of his favorite songs.

- Write a loving, affectionate, sexy note and leave it where he'll find it.

- Send him a spontaneous text message or e-mail that says you're thinking of him.

- Call him but only to ask about him—not to go through your shopping list.

- Offer to run an errand for him and come back with a gift.

- Guide him into a candle-lit bath where you massage his shoulders.

- Compliment him. Tell him, for example, that he looks great—*and make it genuine!*

- Ask him to help you set the table but then reach over, take his hand and give him a smoochy kiss.

- Make breakfast, lunch or dinner in bed for him.

- Surprise him at work with a lunchtime picnic.

- Ensure your next dinner is candle-lit with soft music—even if it's pre-packaged food.

- Don't neglect him; tell him you love him spontaneously. The list is endless . . . And he should be doing these, too!

Don't forget: Some things should be kept private. Cutting your toenails, plucking your nose hairs, going to the toilet (unless you're both liberated about these things!), flossing your teeth, and so on, should be done when your lover's not around. It's hard for him to see you in a romantic light if you're crouched over the toilet seat hacking away at tough toenails!

Other Dating/Relationship Blind Spots

When it comes to dating and relationships, women have many potential blind spots. Here are a few I come across frequently.

What a man says and what he means Men view the goal as more important than the game so they often say things in a way that makes the point without all the detail and honesty. For example, "You're too good for me," means, "I'm too good for you." "It's too soon after my ex," means, "I still love my ex." "I'm not looking for a relationship," means, "At least—not with *you*."

Stereotyping We humans are quick to stereotype. We meet so many people it's easy (lazy!) to slot them into boxes. So we meet a man who seems "shy" and don't give him another chance. What we don't know is that, with a little encouragement, he can be the life and soul of the party. Or we judge a man by his taste in clothes. Many men could benefit from the help of a good woman when it comes to dressing. So, within a few months he could look fantastic if he just had you to bring his style up to date. That's one thing you're allowed to change!

Missed chances Again, I'd be rich if I had $1 for every time a woman told me she missed a chance to go out with someone either because she felt nervous when he asked her out or she was having a "bad hair day" and didn't believe he meant it. Go for those chances when they come along.

Tantric Techniques— So Much More Than Just Sex!

I've included this here, rather than in the "sex" section, as Tantric practitioners are right to say that Tantric practices are so much more than just sex. Tantra says it's *the journey* you take together that's important, rather than the end. So with sex, orgasm is not the goal, it's enjoying the touching and being together beforehand that counts. Tantric principles are about connecting at all levels together. Here are some Tantric practices to try:

- Tantric breathing. To get in tune with your partner, sit facing each other cross-legged. Both of you place your left hand on your own heart and place your right hands on the other's heart. Close your eyes and relax. Eventually, you'll be breathing in synchrony. At that point, open your eyes and enjoy the intimacy of gazing at each other.

- Free your mind of fantasy and simply *feel* the moment together. As you touch each other, let your fingertips, lips and bodies, simply revel in the moment. You should not be focused on orgasm.

- Whole body orgasm. Open your mind to approaching sexual release with a new attitude. *1.* As your excitement rises, let your breathing *relax*—this is the opposite of what we normally do by breathing more quickly. *2.* Clear your mind so that it becomes a blank slate. *3.* Allow your muscles to relax—again the opposite of what we normally do when excited. *4.* Keep moving together slowly and sensually. Gaze at each other and drift into orgasm, allowing all your sexual energy to flow through your relaxed body and breathing.

Babies and Relationships

Many women are shocked to find that their once rampant partner seems to go "off" them after having children. He still lusts after women on TV but doesn't seem to want sex *with her*. This doesn't mean he treats her badly. But what he may have is the "mother-lover" complex. I'll outline this phenomenon as I've heard so many women describe it.

What happens to some men after the baby's arrived is they can only see her in the role of "mother." Somehow he feels it "tarnishes" the mother of his children to see her as sexy. Usually this happens with men from traditional families who tend to look at sex as something naughty. It can be very painful for a woman to suddenly be seen in one-dimensional terms. Try separating the two roles—parent and lover. Agree to no "baby-talk" when it's your "adult time." Whatever you do, don't mention the children. Make a point of acting like you did in the years BC—before children. Start with romance and affection to rekindle things. This can be worked out!

Of course, the reverse is also true and sometimes women feel so overwhelmed by their role as mother that they've nothing left over to give to him as a lover. A woman may not like being touched when she's had a baby at her breast or clinging to her all day. Again a slowly, slowly approach helps. A couple finds that once they're getting more sleep, and adjusting to being parents, things will improve. However, if the problem persists, you should get checked for possible post-natal depression.

How to Argue Constructively

There are arguments in all relationships. Some people argue in a way that doesn't permanently damage their relationship. Try these methods:

- Sit down when calm and identify "hot spots" that make you both angry. Most arguing forms a pattern around a couple of core issues. Plan how to sort out your differences.

- Write out both sides' points of view. See if there's middle ground you can reach and, if so, try planning for these. For example, if finances cause arguments see how your money can be managed so that you're both happier.

- Agree that on some topics you may not reach an ideal compromise but that this may be the best you can do—*so stop arguing!*

- If an argument starts despite following these points, count to ten before yelling anything. Counting to ten works! It gives your brain a chance to get in gear rather than be dominated by passionate emotions.

- If you feel yourself losing control, leave the room, saying, "I'll be back when I'm calmer." It's better to remove yourself when getting out of control than trying to stick it out. But don't use "leaving" as a non-verbal threat to your partner—that you won't be back until you're good and ready—that's unfair.

- Never make sweeping generalizations such as, "You *never* help me!" It's very rare that someone "never" does something or "always" does something. Avoid such statements as they put the other on the defensive.

- Rather than shout, "You f**king b**stard!" try something silly like, "You big dufus!" to dispel some anger.

Domestic Violence

The number of women who experience some sort of domestic violence is staggering. Some estimates put it at one in eight. Most women think, "That'd never happen to me," but it's surprising how domestic violence cuts across class and education barriers.

Often the woman is unaware that the relationship is heading that way as it can creep up in an insidious fashion. The man slowly isolates a woman from her friends and family. In this way he gains control over her ability to do things for herself. She also begins to doubt herself. Or it can happen abruptly: the relationship has seemed "just fine" and then he suddenly attacks her. Often such a surprise attack leaves a woman reeling with fear, and feeling ashamed—so much so that she keeps it to herself. He may be very apologetic and blame it on a particularly stressful period. Any way it begins, domestic violence severely damages a woman's self-esteem. She may begin to believe that she deserves this behavior. It also puts her health—and life—at risk.

Let me make this absolutely clear—no relationship should be based on fear. And an emotional bully can have just as devastating an effect as a physical one. No woman should feel threatened or menaced by her partner. And she should NEVER tolerate violence. If you find yourself in this situation and fear you can't talk to friends or family, call the National Domestic Violence Hotline (800-799-7233) or contact your local police station's domestic violence unit. If events overtake you, simply take your children (if you have any) and *leave* a violent situation. There are refuges around the country and the police will ensure you get to the nearest one that has room. Please do not feel that it's "too late for you" and that you can't leave—you can.

Toxic Relationships

Sometimes we stick in a relationship that is well past its sell-by date. Usually we do this because we refuse to believe the "proof" that we're unhappy. Instead, we cling to the myth that a little more love will change it. Optimism is great—but, at some point, if the relationship is bad for us, we have to face reality. Consider these:

- Do you feel undermined by your partner? Does he put you down in public and/or in private? Does he generally disrespect you? Some men act as if they really don't like women—and look for women willing to put up with their misogynistic behavior.

- Does your partner have an alcohol, drug or other addiction that he is in denial over? Does he refuse to believe he needs treatment? Some addicts are no-hopers who'll never accept their problem. Others need a sharp shock—like a break-up—before they see sense. Once they've sought help, the relationship may pick itself back up and might work. If you have children with an addict you may be willing to take him back if he's getting proper help. But only if he's changing.

- Do you repeatedly argue over the same things, but never solve anything. Have you tried everything—yet your relationship never changes? Some people are gluttons for punishment and never leave unhappy relationships. You do have a choice.

- Does your partner repeatedly cheat on you? Do you keep taking him back? If you want this for the rest of your life—stay with him! If not, trade him in.

Knowing When to Let Go in Love

If your man is "toxic" (bad for you), you can often change his bad behavior by setting your boundaries so he knows he can't cross certain lines. But if you find a man repeatedly fails to treat you with basic respect and kindness, you need to let go. We all have different tolerance levels for bad behavior. You may accept a boyfriend who's a bit bossy because he's got other great qualities and he does accept your point of view if you stand up to him. But frequently we hang on too long. We're often frightened of saying, "I've done my best and this relationship doesn't work." If you're coming to the point of no return, try these final suggestions:

1. Make a note of some examples of his unacceptable behavior—toxic men have short memories.

2. Choose a time when neither of you is short of time or upset over something else.

3. Avoid offering alcohol—you may think it'll relax you both, but it also loosens tongues to say regrettable things!

4. Preface your conversation with, "I think it's time to talk over some problems between us." This doesn't put all the blame on him—quite frankly, you must share the blame for giving him repeated chances to behave badly.

5. Run your examples past him without accusing "You did this...You did that." Simply spell them out factually. Ask for his thoughts on these examples.

6. Finally, tell him this is his last chance to shape up—and mean it. If you back down, he'll always know you'll tolerate his bad behavior.

If none of these work then let go of the relationship!

How to Spot a Liar

Humans tell little white lies all the time—these simply smooth the path of social interaction. For example, you may be late for something and blame it on public transport rather than admit you were dying for five extra minutes in bed. However, some people become chronic liars and manipulators of the truth—they make very bad lovers—and friends! What to watch out for:

- Practiced liars may sit very still (*not* squirming in the chair) but look for tell-tale foot-shaking or finger-tapping as your conversation progresses.

- Liars often latch straight on to your gaze, rather than looking away shiftily.

- Watch out for pupil dilation and lots of blinking.

- As they speak, their voice may literally "catch," almost like a small choking sound—they're literally choking on their lying words!

- Watch for defensive body language, such as crossing their arms behind their back, or across their chest, and leaning back—they're trying to back away from the conversation.

- Liars embellish with lots of detail—too much detail that they really don't need to give. Often it sounds impersonal—like it didn't happen.

- Listen to see if the pitch of their voice rises as they tell their story.

- A lying lover may over-do the innocent puppy dog look.

- They may pause at the start of an answer (as they think of an excuse) and at other points as they continue making up the "facts."

- They may get angry with your questions as their tension mounts.

- Watch for their eyes flicking away with each answer—a sign of discomfort.

- They may answer your question with a question to deflect attention.

The "F" Factors—
Predicting Whether It'll Work

I devised the five F factors to help predict whether your love will survive. They're based on the five areas people talk to me most about in finding harmony/compatibility or disharmony/incompatibility. Think about how these may affect your relationship:

Family background   Research shows that background plays a large part in determining relationship success. If you have similar upbringings you're more likely to have similar outlooks. Opposites can attract but look closely and you may be surprised at the similarities. I'm an optimist and believe love can overcome wide differences in upbringing.

Friendship circle   If you get along with each other's friends your relationship will be easier. But it's possible to tolerate each other's friends for the sake of your relationship, even if they're not *your* choice of best friends. This goes back to respecting the other's choices (within reason!).

It's healthy to strike a balance between spending time together with friends you both enjoy, and separately with friends you both like individually.

Fascination or—let's be honest—the "Fuck factor"! Being amorous with each other at the beginning is easy! Where problems begin is when, for whatever reason, you stop being as hot for each other. Keeping the romance going, and trying the variety of sex techniques outlined in Part One: "Make Love All Night..." will keep things lively.

Financial agreement Arguments about money feature in something like 30 percent of divorces. It's vital that if you have different outlooks you must compromise and *plan*.

Fun and leisure It's fine to have separate hobbies, interests and sports. However, the couple that "plays" together tends to stay together. Find at least one shared interest!

Breaking Up Is Hard to Do

If it all goes south and you're left facing a break-up there are eight key points to remember:

1. You can remain friends but you *don't have to be*. Being "friends" after a break-up is some people's idea of hell, while others see it as incredibly important. Work out what suits you.

2. Expect the unexpected. One day you may feel angry about your ex, the next incredibly sad. Go with the flow and act appropriately, for example, if sad, call a friend and don't isolate yourself.

3. Do something you always wanted to do but couldn't because your ex didn't want to. By doing something new you'll realize that you don't need your ex by your side.

4. Don't become what I call a "break-up bore"—talk about your ex all the time and you'll think about him all the time. So talk about other things!

5. Don't look for love for at least six months. Dating is fine but rebound relationships can be disastrous for your healing—adding a whole other set of problems into the equation.

6. Care for yourself. Be aware of what gets you down—like your "old song." Switch off the radio when it comes on. Remove reminders so that you can move on.

7. Try to put things in perspective. You will love again. You probably loved before this relationship so why won't it happen again? Just don't worry about it.

8. Don't get involved in risky forms of revenge. The best revenge is to get on with life!

About the Author

Dr. Pam Spurr is a psychologist, award-winning radio-show host, national newspaper columnist and a sex advisor renowned for her full and frank advice. She is also the author of *Naughty Tricks & Sexy Tips*, *The Dating Survival Guide*, *The Break-up Survival Kit*, and *Dreams and Sexuality: Interpreting Your Sexual Dreams*. A native Californian, Dr. Pam now lives and works in London, England, making frequent visits to the United States.